GENETIC COUNSELING
Psychological Dimensions

GENETIC COUNSELING
Psychological Dimensions

Edited by
SEYMOUR KESSLER

Genetic Counseling Program,
Health and Medical Sciences Program
University of California, Berkeley
Berkeley, California

With a Foreword by Charles J. Epstein

ACADEMIC PRESS   New York   San Francisco   London

A Subsidiary of Harcourt Brace Jovanovich, Publishers

ACADEMIC PRESS, INC.
111 Fifth Avenue, New York, New York 10003

United Kingdom Edition published by
ACADEMIC PRESS, INC. (LONDON) LTD.
24/28 Oval Road, London NW1 7DX

Library of Congress Cataloging in Publication Data

Main entry under title:

Genetic counseling.

Includes bibliographies.
1. Genetic counseling--Psychological aspects.
I. Kessler, Seymour. [DNLM: 1. Genetic counseling--
Psychology. QZ50.3 G3243]
RB155.G373   362.1'9'6042   78-87879
ISBN 0-12-405650-4

PRINTED IN THE UNITED STATES OF AMERICA

79 80 81 82   9 8 7 6 5 4 3 2 1

Contents

12   Genetic "Russian Roulette": The Experience of Being "At Risk" for Huntington's Disease   199

Nancy Sabin Wexler

13   Genetic Counseling and Cancer   221

H. T. Lynch, Patrick M. Lynch, and Jane F. Lynch

List of Contributors

Numbers in parentheses indicate the pages on which the authors' contributions begin.

Ray M. Antley (115), Director of Medical Genetics, Division of Medical Genetics at Methodist Hospital of Indiana, Inc., Department of Medical Genetics at Indiana University, Indianapolis, Indiana 46202.

John Beck (167), Department of Psychiatry and Behavioral Sciences, The Johns Hopkins School of Medicine and Hospital, Baltimore, Maryland 21205.

Stanley E. Fischman (153), Los Altos, California 94022.

Rose Grobstein (107), Department of Pediatrics, Stanford University Medical Center, Stanford, California 94305.

Verle E. Headings (185), Departments of Pediatrics, Child Health, Genetics, and Human Genetics, Howard University, Washington, D.C. 20059.

Seymour Kessler (1, 17, 35, 53, 65), Genetic Counseling Program, Health and Medical Sciences Program, University of California, Berkeley, Berkeley, California 94720.

Andrew Klein (167), Departments of Psychiatry and Behavioral Sciences, and Department of Pediatrics, The Johns Hopkins School of Medicine and Hospital, Baltimore, Maryland 21205.

Jane F. Lynch (221), Department of Preventive Medicine/Public Health, Creighton University School of Medicine, Omaha, Nebraska 68178.

Patrick M. Lynch (221), Department of Preventive Medicine/Public Health, Creighton University School of Medicine, Omaha, Nebraska 68178.

Henry T. Lynch (221), Department of Preventive Medicine/Public Health, Creighton University School of Medicine, Omaha, Nebraska 68178.

John Money (167), Department of Psychiatry and Behavioral Sciences, and Department of Pediatrics, The John Hopkins University School of Medicine and Hospital, Baltimore, Maryland 21205.

Sylvia Schild (135), School of Social Work, California State University, Sacramento, California 95819.

Nancy Sabin Wexler (199), Commission for the Control of Huntington's Disease and Its Consequences, National Institute of Neurological and Communicative Disorders, and Stroke, National Institutes of Health, Bethesda, Maryland 20014.

Preface

This book deals with the psychosocial aspects of genetic counseling. In contrast to the diagnostic and technological facets of genetic services, or even its ethical and legal aspects, psychosocial issues have been relatively neglected. Over the last few years, however, geneticists have become increasingly aware of the ubiquitousness of psychosocial issues in genetic counseling. The need has grown for a greater understanding of these issues and of the psychological processes by which the aims of genetic counseling are accomplished. This book addresses itself to these various issues and processes.

The book is based on two premises: first, genetic counseling deals with human behavior and psychological functioning; and second, a strong kinship exists between genetic counseling and other areas of personal counseling. Irrespective of how genetic counseling is conceptualized or defined—as an arm of eugenics philosophy, as a communication process, as an information-providing service, as preventive medicine, or as a mental health activity—we are dealing with human actions, attitudes, behavior, beliefs, fantasies, values, and wishes concerning health, procreation, and parenthood. Attempts to educate or inform the counselees about these matters are simultaneously attempts to modify attitudes and/or beliefs, cognitive schemata, and the intellectual understandings, and have an implicit goal of influencing the person's behavior. Likewise the worthwhile, or be it difficult, aim to relieve guilt implies that an attempt is being made to alter the person's effective and cognitive functioning so that behavior is more "effective" and the person feels "better." Thus, as an educator, as a facilitator of decision making, and, overall, as a helping professional, the genetic counselor functions in ways similar to those of other professionals engaged in counseling or psychotherapy. This kinship between genetic counseling and other forms of personal counseling implies that regardless of the specific concerns or problems being considered, the underlying processes and principles are the same. In fact, it can be asserted that there is a connectedness and an underlying unity in all human encounters between a helper and a person or persons seeking help. This unity suggests that where the issues and problems of genetic counseling intersect with those of counseling and psychotherapy, clinical and research data are available to provide us with guidance and direction in our work. Indeed, many of the problems and issues of genetic counseling— Who should counsel and when? How directive or nondirective should the counselor be? What role does the counselor's values and beliefs play in determining counseling outcome? How should the outcome be evaluated?—are already familiar ones to the worker in the field of mental health. A fund of knowledge already exists about these issues and has direct applicability to the genetic counseling situation.

The approach taken here is an eclectic one, reflecting my personal interests and training. It is somewhat biased toward psychodynamic formulations. However, I have not hesitated to draw on other theories (as, for example, systems theory) and on models drawn from cognitive or existential psychology where I felt these formulations were more pertinent to the genetic counseling situation than more traditional approaches.

This book is divided into two major sections. In the initial chapters the principles of genetic counseling are explored, and an attempt is made (in Chapter 5) to integrate these with specific counseling practices. The second section consists of eight chapters dealing with representative genetic disorders. Each contributor was invited to deal with the psychosocial issues related to a specific genetic disorder, or, in one case, the amniocentesis procedure, and, if possible, to suggest specific interventions pertinent to the genetic counseling session. I do not always agree with everything the contributors say or suggest, and I expect that many readers will react in a similar way. The viewpoints expressed in this book are varied—so much so, that the reader seeking consistency or dogma is bound to be disappointed. The fact that such attitudinal diversity exists reflects the overall complexities of genetic counseling itself. There is little in the field (save, perhaps, the genetic fundamentals), about which total or near total concordance of opinion exists. And perhaps this is as it should be for an evolving field that is attempting to deal with multifaceted human questions that have few unambiguous answers. The challenge for the field is whether this diversity of viewpoints can be maintained and nurtured over the years ahead.

Primarily, the book is intended for practitioners of genetic counseling. This comprises a variety of different professionals, including pediatricians, obstetricians, and other physicians; genetic associates; clinical psychologists; social workers; public health nurses; and others involved in the delivery of genetic services. Workers in the general area of medical counseling or health psychology may find the book especially valuable. Medical students and graduate students in the fields of genetics, nursing, social welfare, and clinical or health psychology may also find it useful in understanding the psychological foundations of genetic counseling and in preparing themselves for careers in health settings.

Acknowledgments

In writing this book I have received invaluable help from many persons. In particular I wish to thank my wife, Hilda, for her patient reading of several drafts of my chapters, for her constructive suggestions, and for the many hours of intense discussions which led to a refinement of my own thinking. I wish to thank, too, Nevitt Sanford for his encouragement. Also, I wish to express my gratitude to Doris Gilbert, who read earlier versions of the text and provided helpful criticisms and suggestions as well as constant support. Thanks are due also to Howard Cann and Luigi Luzzatti for their support, and to Clifford Barnett for his suggestions and help. I am especially grateful to Charles J. Epstein for reading the entire manuscript, sharing his insights and suggestions, and writing the Foreword. I wish to thank, too, Adrienne Juliano and Shirley Ross for typing earlier drafts of the manuscript, and Claudia Madison for typing the final copy. Finally, I wish to express my gratitude to the clients and counselees who taught me so much.

Foreword

A few years ago, in a lecture on the present status and future prospects of genetic counseling (Epstein, 1975), I had occasion to review several definitions of genetic counseling, some of which I had either written myself or participated in writing. In a talk given in 1972, I stated that:

> Genetic counseling is the science—and the art—of preventing genetic disease. So defined, the term included not only the more conventional types of counseling . . . but all procedures which lead to the elimination of genetic disorders.

A similar concept was set forth, more succinctly, in the introduction of an unpublished textbook chapter on medical genetics written shortly thereafter:

> The principal purpose of genetic counseling is the prevention of genetically determined disorders. This is usually accomplished by the provision of information concerning risks of occurrence or recurrence.

And, on yet another occasion I wrote:

> Genetic counseling is the process of providing information about the risk of occurrence and recurrence of genetic disease and, when appropriate, of taking steps to modify these risks. Counseling has both a passive component—the giving of risks—and an active one—the modification of these risks [Epstein, 1973].

In all of these definitions there is a twofold emphasis, one on the provision of information—usually in the form of risk figures, and the second on the prevention of genetic disorders. Although the text accompanying all of these definitions included a discussion of the psychological aspects of genetic disease and of the counseling process, it is clear, in retrospect, that the two objectives just mentioned were the major ones.

Contrast, now, the three definitions set forth above with two others. The first is from a World Health Organization report on the prevention, treatment, and rehabilitation of genetic disorders:

> The role of the genetic counselor should be to assist the physician with diagnosis, to estimate the recurrence risk, to interpret this information to the patient in meaningful terms, and to help the patient to reach and act upon an appropriate decision [WHO Scientific Group, 1972].

A new element is introduced by this definition, that of helping the patient decide what to do with the information that is provided. This element is greatly amplified in the final definition, one devised by a large committee of American and Canadian physicians and scientists:

> Genetic counseling is a communication process which deals with the human problems associated with the occurrence, or the risk of occurrence, of a genetic disorder in a family. This process involves an attempt by one or more appropriately trained persons to help the individual or family (1) comprehend the medical facts, including the diagnosis, the probable course of the disorder, and the available management; (2) appreciate the way heredity contributes to the disorder, and the risk of recurrence in specified relatives; (3) understand the options for dealing with the risk of recurrence; (4) choose the course of action which seems appropriate to them in view of their risk and the family goals and act in accordance with that decision; and (5) make the best possible adjustment to the disorder in an affected family member and/or to the risk of recurrence of that disorder [Ad Hoc Committee on Genetic Counseling, 1975].

In this definition there is no mention of the *prevention* of genetic disease. The emphasis is now on *counseling*—"a communication process . . . to help the individual or family comprehend . . . appreciate . . . understand . . . choose . . . act . . . make the best possible adjustment."

There are many reasons for the shift in emphasis from prevention to communication. These include the realization that, certainly in the reasonably foreseeable future and probably in the long range as well, prevention of all or even most genetically determined defects is an unattainable goal—either for theoretical or practical reasons. Furthermore, not all individuals at risk of transmitting a genetic disorder, particularly a relatively mild one, are anxious to prevent its occurrence. While the prevention of a genetic disease or defect might in many instances appear to be desirable to the counselor, it is by no means certain—and we have seen many cases to prove the point—that persons at risk will always be of the same opinion.

Conversely, even if a family or patient is willing to accept prevention of a genetically determined defect as the primary reason for obtaining genetic counseling, the need for sufficient and appropriate counseling cannot be underestimated. This has been forcefully emphasized to me by the results of inquiries made to women (as well as to their husbands) who had undergone therapeutic abortion after the prenatal diagnosis of chromosomal or metabolic abnormalities or the male sex when the woman was a carrier of an X-linked disease (Blumberg, Goldbus, & Hanson, 1975). There is no question that this group was as greatly interested as anyone, including the counselors themselves, in seeking to prevent the birth of a genetically abnormal child. Yet, severe post-abortion depressions were the rule, and serious tension between the marital partners, sometimes leading to temporary separations, was not infrequent. In retrospect it is clear that the amount of counseling required, at all stages of the process, is considerably greater than any of us would have anticipated, and that prevention of disease is not enough.

Last in the list of reasons why emphasis on prevention per se has diminished is the realization that very often the problem is not what to do in the future but what should be done about something that has already occurred. While parental concerns are frequently expressed in terms of risk of occurrence and recurrence, the unstated and frequently much deeper concerns center around the affected child itself and the ways in which they, the parents, may have produced or contributed to its problem. Although genetic counselors have, in general, been cognizant of these problems, they have not until recently been aware of what is actually required to deal with them in a constructive manner.

There is no question that the increased emphasis on the counseling aspect of genetic counseling is a healthy and long overdue development. However, this shift in emphasis has had some curious consequences. For example, I have already been told that because I do not possess the appropriate training and credentials in counseling, I am not a genetic counselor at all. A medical geneticist—yes; a counselor—no! There is great irony in this, since a few years ago I gave a talk in which I expressed exactly the contrary point of view; I, a physician trained in medical genetics, was *the* genetic counselor; all others, including those individuals whose training was in counseling and genetics, but not in medicine, were not (Epstein, 1973)! Both of these statements were made in the context of who should be doing what in an overall genetic counseling situation and, I am afraid, reflect the difficulties that attempts to make semantic distinctions can get us into. The critical point is that our understanding of what genetic counseling is has changed markedly in the last few years, and it is therefore important to recognize just what the concept really means.

In a formal sense, the term "genetic counseling" means just what it says, counseling with regard to genetic matters. Understood in this way, the last of the definitions set for above, "genetic counseling is a communication process . . .," is an excellent definition of what is included. However, I feel, even though I was associated with its genesis, that this definition is too restrictive in its connotations. With its major emphasis on communication, it appears to separate counseling per se from the other aspects of what might be called the diagnosis, management, and prevention of genetic disorders, and I do not believe this separation is either warranted or useful. Counseling does not begin after the diagnosis is made—the making of the diagnosis, with the taking of the medical history and the necessary physical and laboratory examinations, are essential parts of the counseling process. The same is true of the taking of the family history or pedigree and of the calculation of genetic risks when these are required. Furthermore, since appropriate counseling requires accurate facts, it is implicit in this formulation that it is the obligation of the counselor or counselors to certify the accuracy of these facts. The counselor must take direct responsibility for the accuracy of the information, whether it is obtained by the counselor or from others. Otherwise, because of the rarity of several of the conditions dealt with and the complexity of many of the laboratory tests that may be required, there is a very real danger that erroneous information will be transmitted.

Another potential danger of the current "communication" definition and heavy emphasis on the psychological aspects of genetic counseling is the establishment of a dichotomy between physicians concerned with genetic problems and "genetic counselors" who, by implication, are not physicians. This dichotomy is quite pointedly set forth in the WHO definition quoted earlier that starts out: "The role of the genetic counselor should be to assist the physician. . ."

Another expression of the same attitude is contained in references in the literature to "genetic counselors" as patient advocates, with the advocacy referred to presumably being directed against the physician.

At present, genetic counseling has become very pluralistic, with many different individuals participating in the process. These include, among others, medical geneticists (physicians or dentists with postdoctoral training in the diagnosis and counseling of genetic disease), basic geneticists (with various degrees), nurses, social workers, and genetic associates or assistants. Some are more concerned with medical and genetic matters while others deal primarily with psychological aspects. However, while it is true that diagnosis still remains a medical task and, at least in more complicated situations, requires the participation of medical geneticists, the psychological aspects of counseling are not the exclusive province of a single group of individuals. All who deal with patients in a genetic counseling situation must be concerned with communication, feelings, and the solving of personal problems—*all* must be genetic counselors.

This book, therefore, is of importance to all who deal with genetic problems and engage in genetic counseling, whatever their backgrounds or specialties.

Despite the considerable emphasis on communication and the psychological aspects of genetic counseling to which I have been pointing, very little of substance has been written on the subject. This volume clearly represents an attempt to focus on the psychological components of genetic counseling and, by so focusing, to educate the counselors and force them to reflect on what they themselves are doing. I do not agree with everything written in this book; sometimes the disagreements are merely matters of style and taste in counseling techniques, but at other times they represent fundamental conceptual differences. However, this lack of complete agreement is not of importance. What is important is that several psychologically oriented individuals with direct experience in working with families with genetic problems have shared their experiences and thoughts with us. As a result, careful reading of this work cannot help but to stimulate all of us to review our own approaches to genetic counseling and to seek ways to improve them.

Charles J. Epstein

References

Ad Hoc Committee on Genetic Counseling. Genetic counseling. *American Journal of Human Genetics* 1975, *27*, 240–242.

Blumberg, B. D., Golbus, M. S., & Hanson, K. H. The psychological sequelae of abortion performed for a genetic indication. *American Journal of Obstetrics and Gynecology*, 1975, *122*, 799–808.

Epstein, C. J. Genetic counseling: Present status and future prospects. In L. N. Went, C. Vermeij-Keers, & A. G. J. M. van der Linden (Eds.), *Early diagnosis and prevention of genetic diseases*. Leiden: Leiden Univ. Press, 1975.

Epstein, C. J. Genetic counseling—past, present and future, In K. S. Moghissi (Ed.), *Birth defects and fetal development, endocine and metabolic factors*. Springfield, Illinois: Thomas, 1974.

Epstein, C. J. Who should do genetic counseling and under what circumstances? In *Contemporary Genetic Counseling. Birth Defects Original Article Series* 1973, *9*(4), 39–48.

WHO Scientific Group, Genetic disorders: prevention, treatment and rehabilitation. *World Health Organization Technical Report Series*, 1972, No. 497, 1–46.

Introduction

1

Seymour Kessler

Genetic disorders occur among nearly 5% of liveborn infants. In addition, there are many genetic disorders which manifest themselves postnatally; some, like Huntington's Disease, have an average age of onset well into adulthood. When all genetic disorders are taken into account, it is evident that a substantial number of persons, perhaps as high as 10% of the population, may, at some point in their lives, seek out or be referred to a genetic counselor. Genetic counseling promises to assume an important position in the delivery of health care. In fact, it has already done so.

Over the past two decades, dramatic progress has been made in developing and improving the technology underlying genetic counseling. Most important has been the introduction of relatively safe and reliable methods of prenatal diagnosis. Fluid and cells obtained via transabdominal amniocentesis can be subjected to biochemical and cytological procedures which permit the relatively accurate diagnosis of the chromosomal disorders and of an ever-growing number of genetic diseases.

Important changes in legal and social attitudes toward contraception and abortion have accompanied these advances in medical technology. Increasing numbers of couples are seeking assistance in family planning and in ensuring the birth of healthy children. In this regard, genetic counselors have played a prominant role in providing laboratory and diagnostic skills, as well as personal counseling and advice.

While our technical knowledge has expanded, our understanding of the psychological and social implications of this knowledge has, unfortunately,

1

GENETIC COUNSELING
Psychological Dimensions

remained relatively static. The Canadian medical geneticist, Clarke-Fraser has described the psychological aspects of genetic counseling as an area of ignorance and of unmet needs. This is not surprising. From its beginnings in the eugenics movement, genetic counseling was largely divorced from parallel developments in clinical psychology and psychiatry. The polarization of the nature–nuture controversy served to further isolate genetic counselors from the attitudes, principles, and skills of their colleagues in the mental health professions. This historical perspective needs to be kept in mind if one wants to understand the issues and practices of contemporary genetic counseling.

In spite of its biological origins, genetic counseling has gradually become a more psychologically oriented activity. Recognition of this fact is reflected in the definition endorsed by the Ad Hoc Committee on Genetic Counseling of The American Society of Human Genetics (1975) which stated:

> Genetic counseling is a communication process which deals with the human problems associated with the occurrence, or the risk of occurrence, of a genetic disorder in a family. This process involves an attempt by one or more appropriately trained persons to help the individual or family (1) comprehend the medical facts, including the diagnosis, the probable course of the disorder, and the available management; (2) appreciate the way heredity contributes to the disorder . . . ; (3) understand the options for dealing with the risk of recurrence; (4) choose the course of action which seems appropriate to them . . . ; and (5) make the best possible adjustment to the disorder . . . and/or the risk of recurrence of this disorder [p. 241].

This definition leaves many questions unanswered. For example, what are the boundaries of genetic counseling? At what point might it be said to start or to end? Where do the important diagnostic and treatment aspects of genetic services fit in? Are these part of "genetic counseling" or are they separate processes? If they are part of genetic counseling, then what does *counseling* mean in this case? How does one relate it to what is commonly understood as counseling? Also, in many centers different sets of persons may be involved in the various stages of the genetic counseling process; who, in such cases is the genetic counselor? Obviously, there are no simple answers which would apply to all settings in which genetic services are provided. I tend to view counseling as an activity qualitatively different from diagnostic or technical services even though such services undoubtedly have psychological components. The psychological demands placed on the participants in both situations appear to be different. For example, a passive psychological stance in the counselees is often encouraged or demanded during the provision of technical activities whereas a psychologically active stance is generally required in counseling. In actual practice, it may be difficult or undesirable to separate technical and counseling activities in the delivery of genetic services.

Psychological issues permeate every aspect of genetic counseling. The concerns and problems that bring counselees to the counselor and the services and information the latter provides are all ego-threatening in that the counselees must expose themselves to the risk of being shown to be flawed, imperfect, defective, or abnormal and of having the potentiality of transmitting these "flaws" to their progeny. The basic processes on which genetic counseling rests, namely, communication and decision making, are both psychological in nature. Interpersonal communication always has intellectual, cognitive, and affective components. The fact that it concerns the issues of health and illness and of life and death exacerbates the fact that major emotional components are present in the information transmitted in genetic counseling. How information is acquired, retained, and eventually used by the counselees involves a series of complex, multidimensional processes with major rational and nonrational components; again we are dealing with psychological phenomena, poorly understood ones at that. Decision making involves perception, cognition, motivation, personality, interpersonal dynamics, and other psychological factors. Because the issues of genetic counseling have high emotional valence, unconscious motives, needs, and wishes play a major determining role in the counselees' decisions. Since the latter are unaware of this, counselors need to be especially conscious of these factors, even though they are not uncovered in the course of genetic counseling. Also, *how* counselees are helped to arrive at personally relevant decisions involves issues that strike to the core of the counseling process and raise questions as to how and when the counselor's values, beliefs, and personality are to be used to reach outcomes beneficial to the counselees. Psychotherapists have spent decades studying these issues and questions.

The birth of a child with a genetic disorder or providing a couple with a diagnosis of such a disorder generally triggers a series of responses with which the genetic counselor needs to deal irrespective of when the genetic counseling is provided. Here we are concerned with the subtle thoughts and emotions of counselor and counselees alike. The experiences of psychotherapists who have worked with clients, counselees and patients undergoing major life stresses suggest that such points in the life cycle are important ones in effecting changes in the person's personality and intrapsychic and interpersonal functioning. Thus the genetic counselor's interventions, or lack thereof, may have major long-term consequences for the counselees. In many ways, then, psychological issues are an integral part of genetic counseling. Repeatedly we find ourselves turning to the clinician with psychological expertise for guidance in understanding what is going on in genetic counseling because the models of counseling that have emerged from biology are limited or ineffective as tools for providing such understanding. In many ways, genetic counseling has a greater kinship with health and clinical psychology, psychiatry, social work, and mental health than with biology and genetics out of which the field originally developed.

The aim of this book is twofold. First, a comprehensive approach to genetic counseling will be advanced which is based on psychological principles and which attempts to integrate philosophy, concepts, and techniques. The formulation will incorporate relevant points of view from diverse sources—dynamic, systems, cognitive, and humanistic psychology—and will touch on, to greater or lesser extent, theories of cognition, communication, coping and defense, decision making, family functioning, and personality as well as those concerning the goals of counseling, the nature of man, and of the counseling relationship.

No argument will be made that the formulation advanced here is the only one possible for genetic counseling. Other approaches may also be effective. However, so far as I know, no previous model of genetic counseling has been advanced in which specific practices flow from an explicit theoretical base and in which intrapsychic and interpersonal principles are taken into account.

The second aim is to expand our knowledge of the psychological issues underlying genetic counseling and confronted by genetic counselors in their work. In the initial chapters, the major themes will be presented. Chapter 2 concerns a brief overview of the historical development of the practices and principles of genetic counseling and a glimpse into the frame of reference of the psychologically oriented genetic counselor. How a field which deals intimately with so many emotionally charged human issues could have evolved from biology and remained isolated from clinical psychology and psychiatry for so long a period of time is a matter on which students of the history of science need to ponder. Its origins and its current attempts to adapt to the perceived needs of individuals and groups with genetic disorders provide a source of paradox and of flux that is simultaneously puzzling and exciting to observe and experience.

Chapter 2 also introduces the major psychological issues of genetic counseling. These include the areas of health and illness, procreation, pregnancy, abortion, and parenthood. These issues are treated in an eclectic way, drawing on psychodynamic as well as other viewpoints. Wherever possible, the relevance to genetic disorders is considered; this is a first approximation to the development of a psychology of genetic disorders as distinct from other medical problems.

In Chapter 3, the psychological processes essential to the practice of genetic conseling are considered. These include the processes of communication, decision making, and coping. Views will be presented which may be unfamiliar to some biologically trained counselors but are widely known by family therapists, clinical psychologists, and other workers in the field of mental health. The communication process which occurs between a "more-knowing" professional and a "less-knowing" person or persons has multiple levels regardless of the specific focus of the encounter. Without belittling the importance of the content levels of communication, it is essential to realize that less obvious levels of communication exist which may be the major determinants of what is or is not accomplished in the counseling and, when all is said and done, of what the counselees may take away with them, intellectually and emotionally.

In Chapter 4, the psychological meaning of the counselor–counselee relationship will be discussed. The central thesis of the chapter is that the traditional model of the physician–patient interaction is, generally, inadequate for the genetic counseling situation. In genetic counseling, the usual goals are to promote autonomy and to give priority to individual rather than societal needs. To achieve such goals, the genetic counselor will need to reconcile competing values as well as conflicting personal and professional beliefs and philosophies. For some counselors, particularly physicians, these conflicts may be particularly keen. Trained as helping professionals, they are often eager to take command so as to be able to carry out their helping functions. However, what constitutes "help" in, let us say, reducing a fracture, is not the same as helping a person reach a decision about a matter in which it is unclear what is right or wrong. To apply the helping "techniques" of the former situation to genetic counseling, may defeat the accomplishment of the very goals the genetic counselor would like to accomplish.

Genetic counseling and the delivery of genetic disease services is an attempt to influence human behavior so that informed reproductive behavior occurs. It is hoped that ultimately a reduction in the number of individuals affected with genetic disorders will result. Dangers reside in this attempt, not so much in any Machiavellian maneuvers to manipulate the behavior of masses of persons, but rather in an unawareness, on the part of providers of genetic services, of the enormous power of currently existing behavioral control technology. Genetic counseling, particularly provided by persons without a conflict of interest in the direction of research or disease prevention, may become a frontline for the preservation or enhancement of individual freedom and prerogative.

In Chapter 5, the genetic counseling session itself will be discussed and practical suggestions will be made as to how to deal with some commonly occurring themes. Transcripts of genetic counseling sessions will be used to illustrate various points (e.g., different ways of dealing with the counselees' guilt feelings) and of exposing some of the less obvious, but nevertheless important, issues of genetic counseling. Transcripts allow one to see the process of the counseling unfold and they show what is actually said rather than what one thought or had hoped was said. Examination of transcripts reveals that the content of the counseling is often only a minor part of the complex human interplay which occurs in the session. We tend to be largely unaware of most of what happens in the session and, thus, unwittingly, tend to minimize the influence of unconscious factors in determining the outcome of the counseling. Transcripts are a tool to teach us to be more aware.

In the chapters that follow, several contributors will present their views regarding the psychological issues of specific genetic disorders and genetic technology. The genetic disorders around which the various discussions will be organized sample the different modes of inheritance as well as differential psychological issues throughout the life cycle. There are unfortunate gaps; the X-linked disorders are not directly represented nor are the major behavioral disorders (schizophrenia and the affective psychoses) or other major genetic disease entities such as the neural tube defects (anencephaly and spina bifida) and the endocrine dysfunctions, all of which have major psychosocial consequences. Fortunately, many of the psychological issues encountered in these particular disorders are also found in the genetic disorders discussed here. Thus, although the specifics may be absent, the general psychological issues of all genetic disorders are exposed in the various contributions.

In preparing their chapters, the contributors were asked to address themselves to the major intrapsychic and interpersonal consequences of the particular disorder, the psychological issues involved in its treatment and management, and the main issues dealt with in genetic counseling. Each responded to the task in a different way. Some contributors took a broad view of the issues whereas others focused on specific problems directly related to genetic counseling per se. An attempt was made to retain this individuality in the course of editing.

Rather than group the disorders according to the geneticist's usual typology—recessives with recessives, chromosomal disorders with chromosomal disorders, etc.—a developmental sequence will be used here. Genetic disorders with major psychosocial impact generally later on in the life cycle will follow those disorders with relatively earlier impact. We will begin with a consideration of the issues arising from amniocentesis, a procedure used for the prenatal detection of genetic and chromosomal disorders. In Chapter 6, Grobstein, a social worker with many years of experience working in hospital settings, discusses the psychological issues raised by amniocentesis for reason of maternal age. Grobstein argues that the referral by obstetricians of women for amniocentesis with an explanation that a "simple" medical procedure is involved may be misleading and may promote a sense of disappointment and confusion. Amniocentesis involves complex psychological issues and decisions and, although the absolute rate of abnormalities detected through the procedure is low, the impact on the persons whose fetus is found to have a chromosomal abnormality is so devastating that advance, careful work is needed to prepare them for this possibility. The efficacy of such preparatory work, when the individual needs to deal with decisional conflict or prepare for grieving, is substantiated by both clinical observations and research (Janis & Mann, 1977). Grobstein suggests that the thinking about the decision to abort a pregnancy in which an affected fetus has been detected needs to be initiated well in advance of the fact if the couple is to be left feeling that their decision was the "right" one for them. Couples need to understand clearly prior to undergoing amniocentesis that the results of the procedure may force them to decide to continue or terminate the pregnancy. For many, abortion continues to be equated with wrong-doing, sometimes murder. Thus consenting to the amniocentesis procedure raises the threat that one will need to betray deeply held ideals; for some persons, this thought is sufficient to evoke considerable feelings of guilt prior to the fact. Optimally, the genetic counselor needs to assist couples to reach an informed decision on the subject of abortion in sufficient time before they consent to the procedure so that it can be integrated psychologically.

In Chapter 7, Antley, a medical geneticist, deals with the issues encountered in the genetic counseling of parents with a Down syndrome (DS) child. He describes how parents frequently seek to disprove the physician's diagnosis as a means of averting and denying their experience of having parented a DS child. Once the diagnosis begins to sink in, strong affect often emerges; how the genetic counselor handles these responses may have an important influence on the extent to which the parents will be able to "work-through" their feelings and reach reality-based decisions about future courses of action for themselves and for the child.

Antley is a major proponent of a psychologically oriented genetic counseling. He describes how he goes about providing information and simultaneously responding to the counselees' emotional reactions. Antley strongly believes in the healing potential of the counselor–counselee relationship. He strives to build a trusting, accepting relationship with the parents of a DS child from the initial encounter and attempts to maintain relatively long-term contact with them.

Another genetic disorder, often detected in the newborn period, is phenylketonuria (PKU). In Chapter 8, Schild, a social worker, discusses the psychosocial impact of PKU on the developing affected person and on the family. In contrast to DS, effective ameliorative treatment can be instituted for persons affected with PKU. Schild explores the psychological consequences of such treatment and some of the factors involved in inhibiting its efficacy. Parents who comply with the dietary and medical regimen are simultaneously reinforcing their sense of being responsible for the child's "defect." This tends to lead to avoidance behavior and a laxity with respect to adherence to the medical regimen which, in turn, leads to an increasing sense of guilt. For the affected child, the maintenance of health may be purchased at the expense of a lowered self-esteem, as it may reinforce feelings of being "defective" (Moen, Wilcox, & Burns, 1977).

In Chapter 9, Fischman, a psychiatrist, discusses the psychological problems associated with cystic fibrosis, an autosomal recessive disorder generally detected in early life. Not infrequently, the diagnosis of the disorder follows a period of uncertain suspicion on the part of the parents that something is seriously wrong with their child; the diagnosis may actually bring a temporary sense of relief. The demands of the medical regimen to sustain the life of the affected individual have marked effects on the family's functioning. The daily routine of the entire family may be disrupted, creating an atmosphere of frustration. Financial debts may be incurred which, in turn, may interfere with or require major alterations of personal and family goals. For the affected individual, the disorder promotes a state of prolonged dependency that interferes with the process of psychological individuation and evokes multiple psychosocial difficulties which reinforce a sense of worthlessness and of being a burden on the rest of the family. Unaffected sibs often feel neglected and thus bear resentments and ill-will toward the affected sib, with attendant feelings of guilt.

In Chapter 10, Money, Klein, and Beck describe their clinical experience working with persons with sex chromosome disorders. These are frequently detected in late childhood or early adulthood in connection with developmental delays and abnormalities. Money and his co-workers suggest that relatively long-term supportive counseling or therapy may be needed to help the affected individuals and their families cope with these disorders.

Headings, a medical geneticist, deals with the psychosocial issues raised by sickle-cell disease in Chapter 11. This disorder appears to have a major impact on the individual's self-esteem. The affected person's self-expectations academically, vocationally, and otherwise, are lowered. In turn, fatalistic attitudes develop which further interfere with the capacity to live life to the fullest. One might well imagine that if the individual's self-esteem is low, interpersonal relations would also be affected. Stigmatization and concerns about stigmatization are especially prominent in this disorder resulting in fears and suspicions about the ulterior motives of governmental agencies, researchers, and others. Efforts to raise funds, worthy as they may be, often emphasize the harmful, horrible aspects of the disorder as a means of motivating people to respond charitably. These tactics tend to further stigmatize the affected person and reinforce diminished self-worth.

In Chapter 12, Wexler, a clinical psychologist, examines the phenomenological experience of the person at risk for Huntington's disease (HD). This disorder usually manifests itself when the person is in the most productive years, and generally already has a family of their own. The major fears of the at-risk individual involve intellectual deterioration, abandonment, loneliness, and dependency; these interfere with every aspect of the person's life and "infect" the other family members. Relationships with family members and others are disrupted in profound ways. The at-risk individuals question themselves constantly, "How can I involve them? How can I be a burden on them?" A living death often begins at the moment the affected relative is diagnosed.

Wexler points out that a crucial variable in the at-risk individual's adjustment to their risk is the nature of the earlier exposure to the disorder in their childhood. When the affected parent was able to remain functional in the home and/or the quality of care that was perceived to have been received was good, the later reactions of the at-risk person tended to be relatively optimistic. Presumably, the latter was able to learn that, even if ill, one might still be valued and cared for.

The normal processes of identification are complicated by the presence of HD in a family. Identification with the affected parent may be too dangerous for the child—to be like the parent may mean one will also become ill—and may lead to ambivalence and a fragmented identity.

Abandonment is a recurrent theme in families in which HD occurs. It may sometimes be used as a threat, as for example by an angry adolescent against the parent (affected or at risk) or vice versa. In HD families, such threats are especially emotionally charged. Fears of abandonment may sometimes be well-grounded as affected persons are often deserted physically and/or emotionally by their friends and relatives. The at-risk persons fear that the same will happen to them.

In Chapter 13, Lynch, Lynch, and Lynch deal with the psychological issues involved in the cancers. Cancer has much in common with genetic disease in general. In both, the entire person is experienced as affected and the ability to externalize the disorder is difficult. Because postreproductive persons are frequently involved, the affected individuals know that they may have possibly passed genes to their offspring which might make the latter at-risk for cancer. Thus, the former often bear an enormous sense of guilt, the expiation of which may take the form of denying oneself the medical attention one might actually need. To seek and obtain medical help may reinforce one's sense of guilt (How can I be so selfish and so concerned about myself when my child is also at risk?) and to offer oneself up as a "sacrifice" may, on a magical level of thinking, prevent the child's cancer and thus diminish one's personal sense of responsibility.

Themes

Irrespective of the point of the life cycle at which they become manifest, genetic disorders often have major psychological sequelae. Their occurrence and the threat of their occurrence or recurrence strike at our innermost wishes for personal stability, omnipotence, and our normal narcissistic needs. They invariably attack our self-esteem. In this sense, they might be thought of as narcissistic injuries to which the person often responds with various combinations of shame, guilt, depression, rage, lethargy, and stimulus-seeking. The meaning the affected child has for the parent (i.e., the psychological needs which the parent wished, hoped, or unconsciously expected the child to fulfill and which are now threatened because of the disorder), in combination with the person's own life experiences and psychology of the self (Kohut, 1977), are the major determinants of the particular responses to the occurrence or threat of occurrence of a genetic disorder.

In addition to their intrapsychic consequences, genetic disorders have a major impact on family functioning. The relationship between the spouses is particularly vulnerable. Marital discord, separation, divorce, sexual dysfunctions, including impotency, extramarital relations, and increased drinking are among the responses seen by genetic counselors or mental health workers following the birth of a child with a genetic disorder. To a large extent, the interpersonal responses of parents are contingent upon their individual personalities, past responses to stressful events, the stage of the life cycle of the family, the presence (or absence) of a supportive social system and other important variables. Each couple will adopt a strategy of coping designed to keep distress within manageable limits, maintain a sense of personal worth and maintain relations with significant others. Following the diagnosis of a genetic disease, some couples may appear to act decisively with respect to further reproduction.

However, the rapidity of such responses may give them little time to reflect or experience the distressing feelings evoked by the diagnosis. Thus, such responses often serve defensive functions. Similarly, some parents appear to be "paralyzed" with respect to making decisions about further reproduction after a child with a genetic disorder has been born. In both cases, the genetic counselor needs to provide a sense of perspective so that decisions can be made by the counselees on the basis of understanding rather than on that of defensive needs.

Each member of the nuclear family is affected by the birth of an affected child or the diagnosis of genetic disease. Years later, the scars produced by the diagnosis of a genetic disorder and, unhappily, sometimes by genetic counseling itself, are sometimes seen by the psychotherapist and/or marriage and family counselor. Unaffected sibs sometimes bear a disproportionate share of the burden of a genetic disorder. I recall having worked with a young woman who had three older brothers affected with Duchenne's muscular dystrophy. In their own reactions to these children, the parents handed over major care-taking responsibilities to their then preadolescent daughter. Understandably, she perceived her responsibilities as an unjust burden, but her resentment and rebelliousness were not permitted expression at home. Eventually, she fled her parents' home into an early marriage, in which she continued to play the caretaker role, this time to a drug addict.

Another theme associated with genetic disorders is that of guilt and its alleviation. A more profoundly core response to genetic disorders than guilt is that of helplessness. In fact, guilt is sometimes used by the person to defend against an underlying sense of helplessness and powerlessness (see p. 84). Helplessness emerges over and over again in different guises and at different times in relation to genetic disorders. The fatalism of the woman who is convinced that *her* fetus will be the *one* in 800 with DS, the responses of the couple who have been informed that their infant has a genetic disorder, the feelings of the parents who need to bring their child to a *crippled* children service or a birth *defect* clinic for a diagnostic workup or treatment, the couple who needs to choose between becoming parents of a child with a genetic disorder or violating deeply engrained moral beliefs about the sanctity of human life and the parents who through daily ministrations to their affected child are painfully reminded that *they* are responsible for what is happening to their child—all of these are associated with a sense of helplessness which stands in sharp contrast to the growing prowess, understanding, and control resulting from genetic technology.

Field (1971) has explored the problem of the growing depersonalization, alienation, and estrangement of the patient as a consequence of the introduction of science and scientific technology into medicine. Genetic technology has also exacted its price. On one hand, it has opened pathways of potentiality; for example, parents are freed from the burden of having to give birth to and raise a DS child; on the other hand, the parents must take responsibility for making the choice and bear its consequences. The choices offered by genetic technology, like most important life choices, are filled with moral, ethical, philosophical, and psychological dilemmas which have few easy or satisfactory solutions. Thus, in the process of choosing and taking responsibility for our choices, we open ourselves to the realization of how uncertain and powerless we truly feel and, above all, how alone we are in having to decide which life path to take.

Another theme that emerges from these contributed chapters is the need to move beyond the provision of information and facts in genetic counseling. Frequently, counselees come for genetic counseling for more than a search for facts. They come for help in finding meaning in their experiences with genetic disease. As Frankl (1963) has suggested, man does search for meaning in life. These meanings are highly personal and as counselors we are limited in providing others with their meanings. We can, however, help counselees discover these meanings for themselves, and encourage them to put these discoveries to use in their lives. To *encourage* means that we need to help the counselees find their own inner courage to make the difficult choices they must make.

A note to the reader: One of the major tasks of the genetic counselor is to obtain an understanding of the frame of reference of the other person. In the course of reading this book, readers may be required to do likewise so that they might understand a set of concepts and beliefs with which they might not be entirely (or comfortably) acquainted. The traditions, the ways of conceptualizing problems, the reasearch methodologies, and other important issues differ for the geneticist and for the clinical psychologist or psychiatrist. Two potential hurdles need to be kept in mind, one relating to differences in the technical language of the two fields, the other to differences in the kinds of evidence that form the basis of specific courses of action in research, counseling, and other areas of life.

The jargons of clinical psychology and of genetics tend to be different. For example, the term, "client" appears to evoke vastly different images for workers in genetics and those in mental health. McKusick (1973) suggests that the term "consultand" might be used to describe the person seeking genetic counseling, dismissing the term "client" as having "too commercial connotations." Rogers (1951), on the other hand, writes that:

> the term client . . . in spite of its imperfections of dictionary meaning and derivation, . . . seems to come closest to conveying the picture of this person as we see it. The client . . . is one who comes

> actively and voluntarily to gain help on a problem, but without any
> notion of surrendering his own responsibility for the situation. It . . .
> avoids the connotation that he is sick, or the object of an experiment,
> and so on [p. 7].

The same word evokes, in one case, negative, unprofessional sentiments, whereas, in the other, it is used as a term of respect and implies that the relationship between helper and the person seeking help strives toward parity and equality.

Other simple terms also evoke differential responses: directiveness, genetic, projection, reinforcement, supportive, unconscious, and so on. I recall, with not inconsiderable hurt, the derisive response of a group of geneticists to my use of the term, "significant other," a term commonly used by mental health personnel to designate one's mate. Similarly, workers in mental health tend to react with strong feelings to some of the attitudes of geneticists and to the standard jargon that they use in their discussions of genetic disorders and genetic modes of transmission.

In the course of reading this book, the reader will quickly realize that clinical experiences have, generally, been given priority over quantified data. There are several reasons for this. First, none of the currently available studies of genetic counseling effectiveness or outcome are adequate in separating process and other variables from content ones with respect to their effects on dependent variables. For example, in outcome studies of reproductive attitudes or decisions as a function of the magnitude of genetic risk, other aspects of the counseling (e.g., metamessages or the quality of the counselor–counselee relationship) which might have a bearing on the ultimate outcome have not been taken into account. Thus, available research data are of limited value and need to be interpreted cautiously.

Second, there is a need to demythologize the belief that quantified data are really more informative or valid than the subjective experiences of a trained clinician. This belief is an extension into the domain of human behavior of the attitudes and research methodologies of basic science. Such an extension may be inappropriate and, at best, may yield very accurate information about details, but a false picture of the whole.

Maslow (1969) calls attention to two distinct ways of knowing in science associated with two kinds of objectivity. In both, the aim is an attempt to "see only what is actually there." In one case, there is a split between subject and object; the ideal is a detachment or distancing; the observer is a *nonparticipant*; the relationship is, in Buber's terms, an I–it one, uncaring; the observer witnesses or perceives the truths and is not seen as creating them. In the other approach, there is an active effort to reduce the split between subjects and objects; the ideal is fusion; the observers are *participant–observers*; the relationship is an I–thou one and involves caring; and the observers, in part, create the truth merely by being who and what they are and by doing what they are doing. Both approaches are valid, scientific, and useful in shedding light on the process, practice, and problems of genetic counseling. It would be a sad commentary on our profession if we needed quantified data to prove, among other things, that empathic understanding of the other person is valuable and important, that it constitutes the crux of the genetic counseling encounter, or that genetic counseling itself makes a difference in the counselees' lives. We certainly need more research on genetic counseling, but it would be tragic to limit our efforts with strategies which restrict the scope of inquiry and define data gathered by one approach as necessarily more valid than that obtained in other ways.

One last point. Questions have been raised regarding the necessity of acquiring psychological skills among geneticists (see Macintyre, 1977 and the subsequent discussion). Do geneticists need to "become" clinical psychologists or psychiatrists in addition to their other areas of expertise? The question is reminiscent of H. J. Muller's (1922) famous statement, "Must we geneticists become bacteriologists, physiologists, chemists and physicists, simultaneously with being zoologists and botanists? Let us hope so. [pp. 48–49]." Muller's hope has been more than realized—geneticists have become chemists, physicists, and so on, with profoundly important consequences, not only for the profession but for science in general. Is it outside the realm of possibility that they might acquire the skills of clinical psychologists as well?

References

Ad Hoc Committee on Genetic Counseling: Report to the American Society of Human Genetics. *American Journal of Human Genetics,* 1975, 27, 240–242.

Field, M.G. The health care system of industrial society: The disappearance of the general practitioner and some implications. In E. Mendelsohn, J. P. Swazey, and I. Taviss (Eds.), *Human aspects of biomedical innovation.* Cambridge: Harvard University Press, 1971.

Frankl, V. E. *Man's search for meaning.* New York: Washington Square Press, 1963.

Janis, I. L. & Mann, L. *Decision making.* New York: The Free Press, 1977.

Kohut, H. *Restoration of the self.* New York: Basic Books, 1977.

Macintyre, M. N. Need for supportive therapy for members of a family with a defective child. In H. A. Lubs and F. de la Cruz (Eds.) *Genetic counseling.* New York: Raven Press, 1977.

McKusick, V. A. Introduction. In V. A. McKusick and R. Claiborne (Eds.), *Medical genetics.* New York: HP Publ. Co., 1973.

Maslow, A. H. *The psychology of science.* New York: Harper and Row, 1969.

Moen, J. L., Wilcox, R. D., & Burns, J. K. PKU as a factor in the development of self-esteem. *Journal of Pediatrics*, 1977, 90, 1027–1029.

Muller, H. J. Variation due to change in the individual gene. *American Naturalist*, 1922, 56, 32–50.

Rogers, C. R. *Client-centered therapy*. Boston: Houghton Mifflin Co., 1951.

The Psychological Foundations of Genetic Counseling

2

Seymour Kessler

Genetic counseling is an outgrowth of the eugenics movement. Thus, in contrast to most other areas of personal counseling, genetic counseling has its roots in biology rather than in clinical psychology or psychiatry. This has had a marked influence on its goals as well as its principles and practices.

The original purpose of genetic counseling was to carry out the aims of the eugenics movement, namely, to encourage the reproduction of persons with supposedly superior genotypes and to discourage the perpetuation of the genetically unfit. Initially many scientists were attracted to the eugenics movement. However, as it drifted steadily in the direction of social and political militancy, geneticists began to withdraw from active participation (Ludmerer, 1972). With the rise of Nazi Germany and the grim perversion of genetic and eugenics principles that followed, virtually all reputable geneticists repudiated the eugenics movement. Nevertheless, a residue of eugenics attitudes remained evident in the thinking of many genetic counselors. For example, there is a thin line between the view that genetic counseling represents a form of preventive medicine (Leonard, Chase, & Childs, 1969) or that one of its major purposes is to reduce the incidence of genetic disease in the general population (Carter, 1969) and its original eugenics goals. Although many geneticists do not identify themselves as eugenicists, leaders of the now-revived eugenics movement take a different view and continue to view genetic counseling as the major route for achieving eugenics goals (Osborn, 1973).

Closely associated with eugenics attitudes is the view of the genetic

17

GENETIC COUNSELING
Psychological Dimensions

Copyright © 1979 by Academic Press, Inc.
All rights of reproduction in any form reserved.
ISBN 0-12-405650-4

counselor as the guardian of the human gene pool. As such, the counselor might be prone, when providing genetic counseling, to give priority to perceived societal needs rather than to those of the individual or the individual's family. This might be translated into overt or covert attempts to influence the behavior and decisions of the counselees in a direction consistent with the counselor's own value system. The question as to whether the genetic counselor represents the interests of the individual or those of the greater society is not a simple one. Many genetic counselors argue that the interests of the individual should receive priority (Milunsky, 1975). Nevertheless, most geneticists would also like to see a reduction of the frequency of deleterious genes in the general population. In genetic counseling these two values may come into conflict and compromise the counselor's capacity to remain objective and neutral with respect to the counselees' needs and reproductive decisions. This may be particularly true when the extent of the personal conflict is not wholly in the counselor's consciousness.

The most conspicuous evidence of its biological origins is seen in the predominantly content or problem-oriented practices of genetic counseling. Before genetic counseling became concentrated in medical centers, it was generally carried out in academic departments by biologically trained professionals. It was during this period that the nature–nurture controversy was most intense. Most biologists took a strong nature position whereas most psychologists favored a nurture point of view. Thus, relations between the two camps were effectively thwarted. This inhibited the incorporation of experiences and skills of counselors in related fields of personal counseling and promoted the development of counseling practices conspicuously devoid of a psychological foundation. A style of counseling emerged in which the primary goal was the provision of medical information and genetic facts. The major focus was on content material as answers to questions and as solutions to problems. The counseling interaction was sometimes portrayed along the lines of a couple seeking advice regarding the investment of their savings. For example, Reed (1972) writes, "Genetic counseling is much like investment counseling. The investment counselor gives facts and predicts average expectations from them for the future. [If anything, his] empire risk figures are more ephemeral than those of the geneticist [p. 315]."

It was believed that the questions asked by the counselees (e.g., "Why did this happen?" or "What are our chances that this will happen again?") were to be understood literally and responded to in kind. Also, it was assumed that the human decision-making process was inherently rational and that, if the counselor maintained an objective or rational stance and minimized or avoided the emotional issues introduced by the counselees or by their circumstances, this assisted their decision-making process. The counselees' affects, conflicts and fantasies were conceptualized as distractions or as impediments that somehow needed to be disposed of as they interfered with the counselor's ability to deliver information, facts and statistics.

In recent years, a movement away from the content-oriented approach to genetic counseling has become discernible. Several factors have contributed to this development. First, it has become recognized that the medical facts and genetic information conveyed by the counselor are not emotionally neutral for the counselees. In fact, the circumstances necessitating genetic counseling and the actual delivery of such services are highly emotionally charged. Second, genetic counselors have gradually acquired a greater sophistication regarding the principles and psychodynamics of human behavior. It has become accepted that the psychological responses of counselees are not only normal but often a necessary step in comprehending, integrating, and coping with a medical diagnosis or the content material of the counseling session. Third, there is an increasing awareness of the gaps between the purported goals of genetic counseling and the realities actually achieved. For example, although the communication of information is the raison d'être of content-oriented counseling, data suggest that anywhere from 21 to 75% of counselees either do not remember or understand the information they have received (Sorenson, 1974). Psychological processes are believed to set limits to the degree of success one might expect from a content-oriented approach. Fourth, greater attention is being paid to the hidden agendas with which counselees come to genetic counseling. These may involve marital or sexual dysfunctions and other interpersonal difficulties. If attended to, the counselor enters the arena of psychotherapy; if left unattended, these agendas frequently interfere with the counselor's ability to provide information. Fifth, it has become increasingly evident that genetic counseling may have long range consequences for the counselees and their relationship. Genetic counseling may mitigate or exacerbate already present intrapsychic and interpersonal conflicts. Lastly, it has become more widely accepted that one of the major goals of traditional genetic counseling, that of preventing genetic disease, is not an attainable one. "This unattainability is either a theoretical one resulting from the lack of means of actually preventing the disorder or a practical one resulting from an inability to make existing means of prevention available or from resistance on the part of the persons at risk to their use [Epstein, 1975, p. 112]."

A more psychologically or person-oriented genetic counseling has begun to emerge (Kessler, 1979). This approach starts with the premise that genetic counseling deals with human behaviors, important ones at that:

health and illness, procreation, parenthood, and, sometimes, life and death. It views the problems posed by a genetic disorder as being intimately related to the overall situation of the persons, their ways of solving problems, making decisions, and adapting to life crises. Whereas the content-oriented approach emphasized facts, the person-oriented approach places the focus on the various meanings that facts have for the counselees as well as on the intrapsychic and interpersonal consequences of these meanings. Adherents of a content-oriented approach tend to believe that objective facts (and figures) are the base from which decision and action proceed whereas those more psychologically oriented tend to believe that decisions and actions are based on the subjective understandings and meanings of facts. The former approach fostered emotional distancing on the part of the counselor whereas the latter fosters the involvement with emotional issues. In the content-oriented approach, the counselors functioned so as to underscore their roles as authorities, educators, and, often, directly as advisors or decision makers. In the person-oriented approach, the counselor generally functions more as a facilitator, a guide, and, sometimes as a model.

The values, goals, and the strategies used by counselors of the two approaches may differ substantially. For example, let us consider the timing of genetic counseling in cases were a couple has recently sustained a loss. In general, content-oriented counselors tend to be concerned about the appropriate time to provide counseling relative to the loss. They might assume that if the loss continues to weigh on the person's mind then he or she might be unable to assimilate the factual material they hope to communicate. Since they give priority to providing information, such counselors might delay counseling to a time when the counselees have either "sealed-over" emotionally or have sufficiently worked-through their feelings. Since there are no rules as to how long this working-through might take, or, for that matter, clearcut signs by which one might determine that the "appropriate" point has been reached, the content-oriented counselor may never be sure whether this or that point in time may have been or will be more appropriate to provide genetic counseling. Such counselors always run the risk of the counselees "unsealing" at whatever point they decide to do the counseling. What do they gain? One gain is that the counselors may not have to face the full impact of the counselees' emotionality. Thus, the content-oriented counselors gain emotional distance. The losses are several: The counselors may convey the message that either they have no interest in or do not have the capacity to deal with the counselees' feelings. Thus, from the latter's point of view, the counselors have only a limited degree of effectiveness as helping professionals. They cannot be wholly trusted, certainly not with one's deepest fears and concerns. The counselors also lose out in the opportunity to share with the counselees in a significant human experience and thus impose limits on their own growth.

The person-oriented counselor is also interested in the timing of genetic counseling, but from the viewpoint of the phase-appropriate tasks and issues of the mourning process (see Chapter 3). To such counselors, there may be no inappropriate time to provide genetic counseling if psychological issues are actively attended to, whereas, if they are not, no time is appropriate. One of their goals is to help the counselees understand and integrate their experience. The person-oriented counselors might use factual material as a means to that end and in the service of facilitating the mourning process. The risk of this approach is that the counselors may need to get in touch with their own vulnerability in order to help the counselees. The gain of the person-oriented approach is that the counselors open themselves to the experiences, insights, and wisdom of the counselees and thus grow as human beings. The loss involves the giving up of some of the status and power differences often built into the usual professional–client relationship.

Thus, in many subtle, and, sometimes, not so subtle ways, the person-oriented and content- or problem-oriented approaches to genetic counseling diverge in philosophy, goals, and, on a practical level, in the actual interventions made by the counselor. Most important, the former approach moves away from the eugenics implications of traditional genetic counseling and begins to bridge the gap between the views and skills of professionals in related areas of personal counseling and, particularly, of workers in the field of health psychology.

The Psychological Issues of Genetic Counseling

Genetic counseling is directly concerned with human behavior. Thus, it must be based on a knowledgeable understanding of psychodynamics and of the principles of interpersonal functioning. Also needed is an understanding of the psychological meanings of the issues with which genetic counseling is involved, namely the issues of health–illness, procreation, and parenthood, as well as the complex processes by which the goals of genetic counseling are achieved. At this point, I would like to focus attention on the issues of health and illness, procreation, pregnancy, abortion, and parenthood, particularly as they pertain to genetic disorders, and on the multiple psychological meanings they may have for the counselees. In subsequent chapters the underlying processes and some of the major intrapsychic and interpersonal issues will be discussed.

HEALTH AND ILLNESS

The concepts of health and illness are difficult to define (Engel, 1960). These concepts may have different meanings for the physician, the patient, the statistician, or the hospital administrator. For the individual, health and illness may have differing meanings depending on whether or not the person is sick or healthy, young or old.

Attempts have been made to define health and illness in terms of the adherence to or the departures from statistical norms, from optimum levels of functioning and from known or established functional criteria. Offer and Sabshin (1974) have suggested that health and illness ought to be considered life processes rather than states. Subjectively, however, they are experienced as different states of being.

Health is experienced as an awareness of well-being and of effectance. People experience themselves as if their physical and mental capacities are being used in the service of adaptation to the tasks imposed by the life circumstances and the environment in which they live. Illness, on the other hand, is often experienced as a dis*ease* in which people are aware that their physical and mental capacities are not being used effectively to cope with life tasks. Associated with illness are feelings of helplessness, dependency, and discomfort and a narrowing of one's focus of attention and life goals. Some sociologists have equated health with socially desirable or valuable behaviors whereas illness has been equated with deviance (Parsons, 1951).

Subjectively, health is experienced as part of the self. "Health is experienced as intrinsic, as something that is an integral part of the organism as a whole. Its source is from within, and it does not affect parts in isolation [Shontz, 1975, p. 120]." Illness, on the other hand, is generally experienced as an external force and its effects tend to be confined to the smallest possible area of the person's body or life situation.

Because of the threat illness poses to the integrity of the self, psychological defense mechanisms are evoked to diminish or eliminate the attendant anxiety. For example, the illness is not experienced as belonging to the inner self, that is, it is projected externally. All efforts are brought to bear to disown the threat that the illness poses. In the language we use we distance ourselves from the threat by objectifying and depersonalizing the illness and the symptoms of the illness. Patients regularly speak of diseases and of diseased parts of their bodies as objects apart from themselves (Cassell, 1976). Complete denial or repression of awareness of the illness may lead individuals to avoid obtaining the medical attention and treatment they may actually need.

Illness may be experienced as a loss, particularly of one's self-esteem and security and also as a deprivation of satisfaction and of pleasure from usual physical, sexual, and intellectual activities. These deprivations may, in turn, affect interpersonal relations resulting in actual further losses or in anticipations of such loss with their attendant feelings of helplessness, sadness, loneliness, fears of abandonment, and the like.

For some individuals, illness may be seen in terms of a gain. For the person feeling guilt over some past action, illness may represent a just punishment and hence may bring a sense of relief from such feelings. For some, personal illness may allow one to influence or control others and may thus bring a sense of power. For others, illness may reduce anxieties generated by work, sexual, or social demands and thus may be positively reinforcing. In such cases, giving up the illness may be experienced as a loss.

Some of the determinants of the person's psychological response to an illness are personality and life history, the quality of current interpersonal relationships, the physical environment, the specific pathological process involved, socioeconomic, and other variables. The individual's characteristic ways of coping with life stresses will, in general, be manifested in the way he or she deals with illness (Horowitz, 1976). Persons with an obsessive style of personality may insist on detailed explanations concerning their symptoms, diagnosis, prognosis, and treatment. Suspicious or paranoid individuals may project blame on to others for causing their illness or accuse the doctors and other medical personnel of incompetence. Persons with an hysteric personality style may exaggerate their symptoms and become overly dependent and helpless.

The anticipation of suffering, harm, or other danger associated with illness are generally conditioned by one's prior life experiences (Lipowski, 1969). For example, an individual who is aware of a history of Huntington's Disease in his family and has seen the course of the illness in a relative, may experience greater personal threat when feeling temporarily depressed or when an adventitious tremor develops than a person without such a family history.

Experience with illness during childhood colors the meaning that illness has in later life. For many, childhood illnesses were times when the child received rewarding parental attention and sustenance. For others, illness represented restriction, containment, and punishment. Not infrequently the child may associate illness with disability, disfigurement, and death, and sometimes, as a punishment for "bad" actions, wishes, or thoughts. During the oedipal period, the child may experience this punishment in terms of castration anxieties. Because the child depends upon others for caretaking, the sick child sometimes experiences fears of abandonment.

In general, illnesses and the concerns about becoming ill are triggers for

evoking responses, emotions, and feelings associated with childhood. Some
of the attitudes, beliefs, and feelings of this period re-emerge in the
sick adult. The illness provokes a psychological regression to earlier modes
of functioning with an increase of dependency, egocentricity, and passivity.
These behaviors have positive, adaptive aspects in that they tend to concentrate the energies of the person inward toward the self so that they
can be utilized in the process of mastering the illness. Also, they tend
to elicit caretaking responses in others.

Most diseases are experienced as ego-alien and thus externalized. Genetic
disorders, however, are experienced as the consequence of internal "causes"
and thus cannot be as readily projected outward. The genes are part of
the self. They are components of physical structures (chromosomes) which
can be visualized and are integral units of virtually all the body cells.
Furthermore, the genes are invested with life-giving force and enormous
powers. They maintain all the physiological and biochemical processes
of life and keep the person intact and functional. If genes malfunction
or are defective, they cannot be localized and contained because all the
body cells of the person have the same genetic makeup. The entire person
is experienced as defective. Genes have come to play the role in the present
century that the soul played in earlier times. Unable to diminish its threat
via projection only increases the frightening powers of genetic disease.

Many diseases can be treated and the person restored to health. The
person knows, however, that the genotype cannot be changed. It is fixed
for the duration of life. Thus genetic disorders are often experienced as
intractable, unalterable, and permanent; the diagnosis of a genetic disorder
may seem like a sentence of doom. The subtlety required to understand
that the functioning of the genotype may be altered by environmental
manipulation (e.g., dietary treatment in PKU) generally escapes many
individuals. Unconsciously, persons continue to experience themselves as
defective. There is a sense of fatalism, a hopelessness about the future,
and a helplessness to alter natural laws over which the individual has no
control. Moreover, the person knows that it is possible to transmit the
defects to children. Possibly, this has already happened. To be responsible
for an innocent child's illness, deformity, or imperfection may generate
enormous guilt in the parents. This is particularly true if the disease is
not transmitted by an autosomal recessive mode of inheritance and thus
culpability can be ascribed to one rather than both of the parents.
Knowledge of the ubiquitous nature of the mutation process, often suggested as a means of mitigating such guilt, generally offers small solace
to the parent.

Like other diseases, some individuals experience the personal diagnosis
of a genetic disorder as a form of liberation. For example, for some

persons who have difficulties in controlling their drinking behavior, the possibility that alcoholism may be genetically determined may relieve them of enormous guilt. It may also provide some alcoholics with hope that a biochemical factor may be discovered that would explain and absolve them of their "weakness."

PROCREATION

There are multiple motivations underlying the decision to become a parent. On one level, there may be religious reasons, a desire to gain in social status or to conform to social norms, a desire for financial gain (e.g., tax exemptions, increase in welfare payments), and other reasons. On other levels, the desire to have a child may be associated with fantasies of being able to live life over again vicariously through one's child or of improving one's relationship to one's spouse. The desire for parenthood might also be viewed as a way of obtaining greater independence and autonomy, or, on the other hand, as a means of increasing one spouse's dependency on the other. A man, unsure of his masculinity or threatened by egalitarianism in sex roles, may want a large family ("Keep 'em barefoot and pregnant") so that his wife will stay home and be submissive. A woman, unsure of her femininity, may want children to reassure herself that she is a potent female. Pohlman (1969) discusses the psychological factors involved in birth planning. He writes:

> People may want children in part because they enjoy the company of children, enjoy interacting with them . . . [Children] . . . can love a parent and provide someone to love. They can be talked with, played with, dominated and controlled. They provide an audience before which a parent can show off; they admire his accomplishments, and make a hero of him [p. 60].

Having children may fulfill dependency needs. Children often provide the parent with feelings of being needed by another person. Through identification with the child, parents may experience their own needs being taken care of through their ministrations to the child.

Psychoanalytic views stress the unconscious needs and motivations which may be gratified through parenthood. Producing a child is conspicuous public evidence of one's sexual potency and virility. It provides a means of achieving some extension of one's self and one's life (e.g., carrying on the family's name). For some it is an expression of competition with or hostility toward one's parents, siblings, or spouse. For others, parenthood fulfills masochistic needs for punishment for having had sexual desires.

In sum, the reason underlying the desire for parenthood are usually complex, and, in many, if not all instances, the motivations are not entirely within the person's consciousness. In the best of circumstances, the needs and motivations of the two persons involved probably contain some conflicting or ambivalent elements. When procreation entails a risk for a child with a genetic disorder, the ambivalence may be intensified. This may be particularly true in situations where the genetic etiology or the recurrence risk is ambiguous. For example, in one couple with a child with a split hand and foot deformity, each subsequent pregnancy was both intensely desired and intensely feared. When the wife was not pregnant, she strongly desired another child. This led to difficulties in managing one form of contraception after another until a pregnancy occurred. Once pregnant, the fear of having another affected child increased which eventually led her to obtain a therapeutic abortion. This process had been repeated three times before the couple came for genetic counseling.

Couples with strong unconscious needs or motives to have a child are likely to understand the information obtained in genetic counseling differently than couples not so motivated. Both sets of couples may selectively attend to certain pieces of information or distort a recurrence risk figure so as to find support for their respective needs. Thus, according to their unconscious needs, the same genetic risk figure may seem negligible to one couple and enormous to another.

PREGNANCY

From a developmental perspective, a couple's first pregnancy is an important milestone for their relationship and for each partner individually. The pregnancy requires the assumption of new roles and identities as parents, which, in turn, requires a readjustment in their relationship to accommodate these roles. For some period of time, the wife may need to be emotionally and financially dependent on her husband. Both partners may have to curtail activities freely engaged in prior to the pregnancy. Adapting to the parental role invariably raises unresolved conflicts from their own childhood and fears concerning their adequacy and capacity to be parents (Hittelman & Simons, 1977).

Pregnancy generally has multiple psychological meanings for the prospective parents. Psychoanalytic writers often view pregnancy as a means of gratifying unconscious wishes concerning penis envy. There appears to be considerable agreement that the meaning a pregnancy has for a woman depends largely on how she feels about herself as a woman. The extent to which she has resolved childhood conflicts with her own mother and the degree to which she accepts and respects her body and her self in general, often shape these feelings (Benedek, 1970b).

How the pregnant woman feels about herself will also influence her feelings toward the unborn child. If, consciously or unconsciously, she experiences herself as deficient or defective, she may imagine that since the child is part of herself, it too is deficient or defective. In other words, her self-image is reflected in the mental image of the child. Conversely, her fantasies regarding the child are projections of the feelings she has about herself.

The prospect of producing an infant with a congenital defect or genetic disorder is entertained by virtually every pregnant woman, and presumably, by every prospective father as well. Pregnant women frequently fantasize or dream about their unborn child and, sometimes the child is seen as deformed or dead. In one's unconscious the person comes face to face with the dreaded projections of one's own unloved or deficient self.

The changing psychological perceptions of the pregnant woman are described by Bibring (1959). In the first trimester of pregnancy, the major focus of the prospective mother is centered on the somatic and physiological change she is experiencing. At this stage, mother and fetus are experienced as one. Quickening initiates a second stage, in which the mother perceives the baby as an object apart from herself. This perception prepares the mother gradually for the delivery and forthcoming anatomic separation between herself and her child.

It is important to note that the amniocentesis procedure is carried out just prior to this crucial psychological stage. Thus, it needs to be kept in mind that commitments or decisions concerning the pregnancy made in early stages may be experienced differently in later stages of the pregnancy. For example, it might be easy for a woman in her twelfth week of pregnancy to agree to a later therapeutic abortion should a prenatal test show that the fetus has a chromosomal disorder. However, once she has experienced the fetus as a separate, active, living being, the contemplation of an abortion may have different meanings and may be difficult for her to actually undergo.

The psychological experiences and effects of amniocentesis are poorly understood and, because it is a relatively new procedure, have not been intensively studied. In amniocentesis, the woman's body boundaries are penetrated. Does this accelerate the differentiation between the self and the prenatal object? Is the experience especially threatening because mother and fetus are poorly differentiated?

The amniocentesis procedure is anxiety-provoking. Invariably, couples are concerned about the safety of the procedure, both for the mother and for the fetus. Dreams reported prior to and just after undergoing amniocentesis appear to be filled with disquieting themes. For example, the following dream was reported by a woman two nights after having undergone amniocentesis:

> I dreamed that I had miscarried the baby. . . . My abdomen seemed to open up quite naturally as if it was a kangaroo's pouch. The baby seemed to come in two Saran bags, one containing the head, one the body. I was distraught that I was about to lose it.
>
> My dream moved into an admissions section of a hospital where I desperately explained the situation. They casually told me to take some codeine which infuriated me and I began to argue very emotionally. I was finally taken to a room on the perimeter of the hospital that happened to be used for storing objects. A janitor was polishing the corridor floor and the doctor asked him to assist. I was told it was too late, the baby was dead. . . .
>
> I then found myself in my obstetrician's office, emotionally describing what had happened (in tears). He tried to console me . . . Finally he told me that it hadn't really happened anyway and that it was just a dream.

Particularly pertinent in the dream is the dreamer's experience of the health care system as being callous and unresponsive to her needs and finally, as having her fears and emotions disqualified by the obstetrician ("it hadn't really happened anyway . . . it was just a dream."). The dream may be seen as anticipatory grief (Lindemann, 1944) for the fetus that she may need to abort if the diagnosis of chromosomal disorder is made. On another level, it is also preparatory work for her forthcoming delivery, in which she indeed will have to give up the baby to the birth process.

Ashton (1976) reports having the following dream the night before undergoing amniocentesis. She writes:

> A friend called me on the night before the test to assure me that there was nothing to worry about . . . I accepted the statement rationally, of course, but when I fell asleep, I dreamt that I was in the hospital being put under ether—the recreation of a childhood scene. A large, spinning wheel was in front of me filled with flashing letters of the alphabet out of which I was instructed to make words. "Biology," I spelled out painfully and then "luck" before I floated away into total unconsciousness [p. 5].

The dreamer informs us that her rational understanding does not mitigate the worry, concern, and apprehension she actually feels. Childhood fears and traumas are reawakened. In the dream she seems to be alone (although another presence is implied) as she experiences the anxiety of waiting for the wheel of fortune to indicate what lies in store.

The dream itself bears a remarkable similarity to the image of card X of the Waite-Smith Tarot which is called the Wheel of Fortune (Waite, 1911). The card depicts a wheel on top of which a sphinx is seated. On the wheel itself are Latin letters spelling out, from 12 o'clock counterclockwise, the word TORA, the Hebrew word for law. Interspersed between each of these letters are Hebrew letters which spell out the Tetragrammaton (JHVH) or the Merciful Name of God. Lawfulness is the province of science in general, including "Biology" whereas the concept of mercy and of divine intervention might be granted with "luck" and chance. Thus the dream exposes both the fears and wishes of the dreamer and, through archetypal symbolism, unites her to the human drama of the life cycle.

One of the fears of many pregnant women is of death in childbirth. Despite the enormous gains of medical science in the twentieth century in reducing such risks, the fear of death during delivery continues to persist. Bibring (1959) suggests that the emotional health of pregnant women is actually undermined by the attitudes of scientific medicine which communicate to women the demand to take an objective attitude toward themselves, the fetus, and their pregnancy.

ABORTION

The psychological aspects of abortion are discussed by Pohlman (1969) and by Senay (1974). Psychotherapists have long known that for many women abortion is a profound experience. Years afterwards, memories of the procedure and of the circumstances surrounding it, may intrude into the woman's awareness. They may still feel pangs of remorse, shame, and guilt, cry for the child that they might have had, and indulge in self castigation. Even when faced with the awareness that given the same circumstances they would probably undergo abortion again, the painful feelings often persist.

Since the wanton taking of human life is culturally reprehensible, most persons have ambivalent feelings regarding abortion. Despite the clinical attitudes taken by many professionals and the attempts to depersonalize the fetus, on one level of awareness, the decision to abort a pregnancy involves the knowledge that one is acting contrary to one's inner moral and ethical values (Callahan, 1970). Abortion is frequently experienced as murder. Yet, given the choice between giving birth to a defective child or aborting, many couples choose the latter. This decision often has profound, long-lasting consequences.

Blumberg, Golbus, and Hanson (1976) studied families in which the woman had undergone amniocentesis and selective abortion following the prenatal detection of an affected fetus or of a potentially affected one in the case of X-linked disease. These workers found that selective abortion had multiple psychological ramifications for a majority of the couples. Almost all the subjects in the study (92% of the women and 82% of the men) showed evidence of depression that appeared to be of greater intensity than the depression generally associated with stillbirths. The self-esteem of many of the subjects tended to be undermined and, because they perceived themselves to be responsible for the abortion, feelings of guilt were intensified. Memories of earlier stresses were reawakened and future difficulties were anticipated. Marital difficulties occurred among some of the couples. Lastly, many women experienced "flash backs" (i.e., intrusive thoughts and emotions associated either with the abortion or with objects and events related to babies and childbirth) long after the procedure.

Blumberg *et al.* also found that feelings of guilt tended to be exacerbated among women who were carriers of X-linked disorders as compared to those involved with recessive or sporadic disorders. In cases where the pregnancy was terminated with a 50% chance of producing a defective child, most couples tended to convince themselves retrospectively that the aborted fetus had indeed been affected. Thus, guilt feelings and doubts concerning the correctness of their decision to abort the fetus were generally subjected to defensive rationalization.

PARENTHOOD

Our past conceptions regarding the family and parenthood developed during a period of history in which the patriarchal model of the family was predominant. The roles of the father and the mother were assumed to be static, and according to some writers, biologically predetermined. Gender related tasks were relatively clear-cut: The father was the provider–protector or instrumental leader whereas the mother was the nurturing or expressive-affective leader of the family (Lidz, 1974). As the roles of the two parents were seen as static, it was assumed that their respective personalities were also set and stable and not influenced by their relationships with the growing child (Benedek, 1970a). This traditional model has come under attack from many quarters, most particularly from the feminist movement. Increasingly, couples are encountered in genetic counseling whose values and beliefs regarding marriage, parenthood, abortion, and the like are divergent from the traditional patriarchal ones. It would be a mistake for genetic counselors to assume that counselees necessarily share the same framework of beliefs regarding these issues as they do.

Family therapists and contemporary psychodynamic views emphasize the developmental aspects of the family and of parenthood. Each partner brings to their relationship his or her own personality as well as attitudes, beliefs, values, and a fund of experience from his or her own nuclear family. If their needs are gratified through their relationship, each partner becomes a part of the self-system of the other. With the birth of the first and subsequent children further opportunities are provided to achieve another level of personality integration (Benedek, 1970a). As the child attains developmental and social milestones (school, dating, marriage, establishment of their own families), each parent has an opportunity to reexperience their own developmental past. Thus, from a different (and more mature) vantage point, the parent can relive childhood fears and conflicts and bring resolution to open issues. The child, then, plays an instrumental role in furthering the developmental integration of the parent. The child is like a mirror in which the parents see reflected back both the positive and negative aspects of their own behavior and personality. "[W]hile the parents consciously try to help the child achieve his developmental goal, they cannot help dealing unconsciously with their own conflicts, and thus, they achieve a new level of maturation themselves [Benedek, 1974, p. 489]."

When viewed from the perspective of the central role the child plays in furthering the normative development and maturation of the parent, one can obtain an understanding of the enormously disruptive effect the birth of a child with a congenital or genetic disorder may have. Instead of the joy, satisfaction, and self-fulfillment provided by the normal child, the parents see their own deficiencies and defects reflected back. One sees the unloved self. The mourning reactions seen in parents following the birth of a child with a congenital or genetic disorder have often been interpreted as a response to the loss of the wished-for healthy child and a gradual decathexis or giving up of the emotional investments in and attachments to this wish (Solnit & Stark, 1961). However, more than the mental image of a healthy child is lost for the parent. Also lost are intuitive potentialities for personal development. Unable to identify with the child, the parent cannot reexperience and rework their own past. In a sense, the parent is cheated from experiencing and participating in an important aspect of the life cycle. Thus, the normal course of maturation is derailed. How long and the degree to which this derailment persists depends on many factors including the ego strengths of the individual, the quality of external support systems, the presence of other children in the family, and so forth. Some individuals convert the tragedy of a genetic disorder into a transcendent experience and achieve personal satisfaction and growth via alternate routes.

Record and Armstrong (1975) found that the death of a baby in the perinatal period or during the first year of life was followed by an increased likelihood of a subsequent birth with a decrease in the birth interval. If the child with a serious malformation survived the first year of life, the parents tended to delay subsequent reproduction and overall had a slightly smaller number of children than might have been expected. Presumably, in the latter case, the increased caretaking demands and the economic and emotional burdens imposed on the family as a consequence of the presence of the affected child diminished desires for additional children.

The various routes chosen by parents to deal with the death of a child early in life may have differing psychological meanings. Compensatory reproduction may be a means of reconfirming one's potency or one's capacity to produce a healthy baby and of dealing with feelings of depression. Not infrequently parents move away to another community following the death of a child. This may be a means of letting go of emotional investments and ties as well as of painful memories. It may also represent a means of dealing with feelings of shame over having disappointed friends and relatives by having produced a defective child to begin with or by having "failed" as parents. Sterilization is another route parents sometimes take to deal with early loss. This may be a way of dealing with guilt feelings of having brought a defective child into the world. Also, it may be a means of punishing one's unloved self and thus expiating guilt feelings.

References

Ashton, J. Amniocentesis: Safe but still ambiguous. *Hastings Center Report*, 1976, 6, 5–6.

Benedek, T. The family as a psychologic field. In E. J. Anthony & T. Benedek (Eds.), *Parenthood: Its psychology and psychopathology*. Boston: Little Brown and Co., 1970a.

Benedek, T. The psychobiology of pregnancy. In E. J. Anthony & T. Benedek (Eds.), *Parenthood: Its psychology and psychopathology*. Boston: Little Brown and Co., 1970b.

Benedek, T. The psychobiology of parenthood. In S. Arieti (Ed.), *American handbook of psychiatry*, 2nd ed., (Vol. 1). New York: Basic Books, 1974.

Bibring, G. L. Some considerations of the psychological processes in pregnancy. *Psychoanalytic Study of the Child*, 1959, 14, 113–121.

Blumberg, B. D., Golbus, M. S., & Hanson, K. H. The psychological sequelae of abortion performed for a genetic indication. *American Journal of Obstetrics and Gynecology*, 1975, 122, 799–808.

Callahan, D. *Abortion: Law, choice and morality*. New York: Macmillan, 1970.

Carter, C. O. Genetic counseling. *Medical Clinics of North America*, 1969, 53, 991–999.

Cassell, E. Disease as an "it": Concepts of disease revealed by patients' presentation of symptoms. *Society for Science & Medicine*, 1976, *10*, 143–146.

Engel, G. L. A unified concept of health and disease. *Perspectives in Biology and Medicine*, 1960, *3*, 459–485.

Epstein, C. J. Genetic counseling: Present status and future prospects. In L. N. Went, Chr. Vermeij-Keers & A. G. J. M. van der Linden (Eds.), *Early diagnosis and prevention of genetic diseases*. Leiden: Leiden Univ. Press, 1975.

Hittleman, J. & Simons, R. C. Pregnancy and the expectant couple. In R. C. Simons & H. Pardes (Eds.), *Understanding human behavior in health and illness*. Baltimore: Williams and Wilkens Co., 1977.

Horowitz, M. J. *Stress response syndromes*. New York: Jason Aronson, 1976.

Kessler, S. The genetic counselor as psychotherapist. In M. Lappé, S. B. Twiss, A. Capron, R. Murray & T. Powledge (Eds.), *Genetic counseling: Facts, values and norms*. Miami, Florida: Plenum Press, 1979.

Leonard, C. O., Chase, G., & Childs, B. Genetic counseling: A consumer's view. *New England Journal of Medicine*, 1972, *287*, 433–439.

Lidz, T. The family: The developmental setting. In S. Arieti (Ed.), *American handbook of psychiatry*, 2nd ed., (Vol. 1). New York: Basic Books, 1974.

Lindemann, E. Symptomatology and management of acute grief. *American Journal of Psychiatry*, 1944, *101*, 141–148.

Lipowski, Z. J. Psychosocial aspects of disease. *Annals of Internal Medicine*, 1969, *71*, 1197–1206.

Ludmerer, K. M. *Genetics and American society*. Baltimore: Johns Hopkins Univ. Press, 1972.

Milunsky, A. Genetic counseling: Principles and practice. In A. Milunsky (Ed.), *The prevention of genetic disease and mental retardation*. Philadelphia: W. B. Saunders Co., 1975.

Offer, D. & Sabshin, M. *Normality*. New York: Basic Books, 1974.

Osborn, F. The emergence of a valid eugenics. *American Scientist*, 1973, *61*, 425–429.

Parsons, T. *The social system*. New York: The Free Press, 1951.

Pohlman, E. *The psychology of birth planning*. Cambridge, Mass.: Schenkman Publ. Co., 1969.

Record, R. G. & Armstrong, E. The influence of the birth of a malformed child on the mother's further reproduction. *British Journal of Preventive Social Medicine*, 1975, *29*, 267–273.

Reed, S. C. Genetic counseling in schizophrenia. In A. R. Kaplan (Ed.), *Genetic factors in "schizophrenia"*. Springfield: Thomas, 1972.

Senay, E. C. The psychology of abortion. In S. Arieti (Ed.), *American handbook of psychiatry*, 2nd ed., (Vol. 1). New York: Basic Books, 1974.

Shontz, F. C. *The psychosocial aspects of physical illness and disability*. New York: Macmillan Publ. Co., 1975.

Solnit, A. J. & Stark, M. H. Mourning and the birth of a defective child. *Psychoanalytic Study of the Child*, 1961, *16*, 523–537.

Sorenson, J. R. Genetic counseling: Some psychological considerations. In M. Lipkin, Jr. and P. T. Rowley (Eds.), *Genetic responsibility*. New York: Plenum Press, 1974.

Waite, A. E. *Pictorial key to the tarot*. London: W. Rider, 1911.

The Processes of Communication, Decision Making and Coping in Genetic Counseling

3

Seymour Kessler

Some of the major tasks of the genetic counselor are to communicate medical information and genetic facts, to help the counselees reach pertinent decisions, and to help them cope with the information supplied in counseling as well as with the consequences of the genetic disorder. In this chapter the processes underlying these tasks will be considered. First, the principles of human communication will be examined. Communication is the *means* by which genetic counseling is accomplished; because of its salience, the process of communication is sometimes mistaken for the counseling process itself. Since effective communication and effective counseling are related, the factors known to lead to effective outcomes in personal counseling will be included in our discussion. This will be followed by a brief consideration of recent research on human decision making. In this chapter, decision making involving the assessment of probability and genetic risks will be discussed. In Chapter 5, the decision-making process will be approached from a different perspective and the subject of how to help counselees make autonomous decisions will be considered. Finally, because genetic counselors frequently see couples in various stages of mourning for a deceased relative or coping with a recent diagnosis of a genetic disorder, the processes subsumed under the term *coping behavior* will be discussed in some detail.

Human Communication

In some respects, genetic counseling is similar to the physician–patient interaction. It differs in two major respects. First, in genetic counseling, most counselees are neither ill nor patients and thus do not require the

GENETIC COUNSELING
Psychological Dimensions

medical attention and interventions generally accorded persons threatened with the loss or curtailment of vital functions. Second, whereas decisions regarding future health are often expected to be made by the physician, in genetic counseling it is expected that such decisions will be made by the counselees (Sorenson, 1973). Despite these differences, it would be illuminating to explore briefly the effectiveness of physician–patient communication before examining the analogous process that occurs in genetic counseling.

Studies summarized by Korsch and Negrete (1972), suggest that considerable shortcomings exist in the communication process between physician and patient. These difficulties are attended by feelings of mutual dissatisfaction and, often, the effectiveness of the health care provided is diminished. Korsch and co-workers observed over 800 visits to a walk-in pediatric clinic and tape recorded a majority of the physician–patient interactions. In this case, the mothers were defined as the patients. Following the visit, these investigators found that about half of the mothers were still not clear as to what had caused their child's illness. An analysis of the content and tone of the verbal interactions revealed that the physicians tended to use medical and technical jargon, which, although it impressed and even flattered some patients, left most of the mothers unenlightened about the nature of their child's illness. The physicians related better with the children than with the mothers. They often disregarded the mother's concerns and discounted her perceptions of the child's illness. Korsch and Negrete (1972) write:

> Among the 800 mothers, 26 percent told interviewers after the session with the doctor that they had not mentioned their greatest concern to the physician because they did not have an opportunity or were not encouraged to do so.
> Under such circumstances there was frequently a complete breakdown of communication. Some patients were so preoccupied with their dominant concerns that they were unable to listen to the physician [p. 72].

Understandably, a majority of the mothers who felt that the physicians had not understood their concerns were dissatisfied with the visit, whereas most of the mothers who reported that the physician had understood them were satisfied. Dissatisfaction was strongly associated with noncompliance with the physician's medical advice. Of the mothers who reported satisfaction with the interaction with the physician, 53.4% cooperated completely with the doctor's advice whereas only 16.7% of the dissatisfied mothers did so.

A detailed study of the communication process in genetic counseling has not yet been reported. Nevertheless, several outcome studies carried out in the United States and elsewhere suggest that, as in the physician–patient relationship described above, difficulties exist in conveying medical and genetic information to genetic counselees. Leonard, Chase, and Childs (1972) studied 61 families with at least one child affected with one of the following genetic disorders: phenylketonuria (PKU), cystic fibrosis, Down syndrome (DS). Each family had received genetic counseling, following which the parents were interviewed to determine their knowledge of the specific disease, of the genetic risks involved and of other biological and genetic information. These workers concluded that only about half "of the parents had the kind of comprehension that could make this information helpful to them ... [p. 436]." Furthermore, they write that:

> some parents who did give correct answers denied their validity or said that they did not apply to themselves. Others confessed to a lack of comprehension of the correct answers that they had given, and some exhibited a lack of perception of the meaning of the risk. Few of the parents of DS children knew what a chromosome is, or could differentiate it from a gene, although these points had been made by the counselor [p. 436].

It is noteworthy that of the 61 families, 5 claimed that they had not even received genetic counseling! In other studies of genetic counseling outcome, it has been reported that between 21 and 75% of counselees fail to remember or acquire the genetic information provided (Sorenson, 1974).[1] Clearly, then, a gap exists between the goals genetic counselors intend to reach and the goal actually being accomplished with respect to the communication of factual information. It is easy to imagine that many, if not all, of the difficulties in communication identified in studies of the physician–patient interaction also exist in the genetic counseling encounter. No amelioration of these problems can occur without a better understanding of the principles of human communication.

Human communication occurs on multiple simultaneous levels (Ruesch

---

[1] The value of outcome studies that assess counselee memory for details of a previous genetic counseling session needs to be questioned. Baseline levels of counselee knowledge have rarely been given by investigators. Thus it is not clear whether most currently available data represent initial levels of knowledge or the effects of counseling interventions. Also the meaning of the findings is obscure. The fact that counselees remember the information provided during genetic counseling may have little bearing on the reproductive decisions made later on. In the decision-making process some information may be selectively repressed or recalled. Also, information not recalled at the time of testing may nevertheless be stored and may contribute substantially to later reproductive decisions.

& Bateson, 1951; Haley, 1963; Satir, 1964; Watzlawick, Beavin, & Jackson, 1967). Two major ones will concern us here, the denotative and meta-communicative levels. The former encompasses the literal content of communication whereas the latter is the route by which the sender conveys messages about needs, feelings, and states of awareness below the level of consciousness. Metacommunications often take the form of nonverbal behavior (e.g., posture, gestures, the way the person breathes). Also, they are expressed in the way the voice is used (e.g., its quality, tone, and volume). Satir (1964) writes that the metacommunication is:

> a comment on the literal content as well as on the nature of the re-lationship between the persons involved . . . It conveys the sender's at-titude toward the message he just sent . . . the sender's attitude toward himself . . . [and] the sender's attitude, feelings, intentions toward the receiver . . . Humans . . . cannot communicate without, at the same time, metacommunicating. Humans cannot *not* metacommunicate [p. 76].

A second major principle of human communication is that in a social setting it is impossible to not communicate. Even a nonresponse to a message is a communication. For example, in some psychotherapy situa-tions, a client's question may be answered with silence on the part of the therapist. This may convey the message, "I ask the questions here, not you."

When individuals experience anxiety, it often affects the communi-cation process. The messages conveyed on the different levels of com-munication may be incongruent, that is, the message on one level may fail to jibe with that on another level. Saying "yes" while shaking one's head "no" is an example of such an incongruency. Incongruencies may reflect the presence of an unresolved conflict. Also, it may be the means by which persons defend themselves from overtly revealing feelings of guilt, shame, or depression.

When a message evokes anxiety in a receiver, it is likely that the per-son's self-esteem is being threatened or that there is an anticipation of such a threat. Often, in such cases, the message is distorted or discounted so as to reduce the threat.

Sometimes messages and metamessages involve such conflicted impli-cations or injunctions that the receivers feel damned if they do and damned if they do not. This is known as a "double bind" (Bateson, Jackson, Haley, & Weakland, 1956). For example, at the end of a tiring session, the genetic counselor might ask the counselees, "You've gotten something out of this session, haven't you?" At least two metamessages may be conveyed: "I've worked hard and I hope you appreciate it," and

"If you feel that you haven't gotten anything from me, I expect you not to say so." Both the sender and the receiver are in a bind. If the counselees respond sincerely, "yes," the counselor may have difficulty believing them because they may only be saying so to protect the counselor's sensibilities. If the counselees respond, "no," they risk the counselor's displeasure as it has already been implied that they should say "yes." All parties lose in a double bind situation.

Another important aspect of human communication is the context in which it occurs. The context includes physical, social, and syntactic components. The fact that most genetic counseling is carried out in medical centers has a major influence on the communication between counselors and counselees. The counselor is on home ground and is generally surrounded by persons and things—nurses, paramedical personnel, laboratories, hospital odors, laboratory coats, and so forth—which have stimuli value for the counselees and generally shape their behavior in the direction of compliance, deference, and cooperativeness. Patients (and, presumably counselees) who fail to behave according to the expectation of medical and paramedical personnel tend to be labeled as aggressive, obstructive, or uncooperative (Gillum & Borsky, 1974). The medical center atmosphere is a familiar one to the counselor; the registration procedures, the corridors, the page system, the hustle–bustle milieu are generally hardly noticed by the counselor. For the counselees, the same stimuli may evoke frightening images (and/or memories) and induce not inconsiderable anxiety, discomfort, confusion, and helplessness.

The social setting also contributes to the communication that takes place in genetic counseling. For example, the same information conveyed by telephone has a different meaning than when conveyed in a face-to-face encounter. In the former situation, the opportunity for physical contact and support between sender and receiver is impossible and the range of emotional interchange is severely curtailed as compared to the latter. The presence of two counselors, one male and one female, may be experienced differently than the presence of either counselor alone. In the former case, the counselees might perceive a message that each will have an ally in and support from the same-sexed counselor. If a differential status is (consciously or unconsciously) emphasized in the male–female counselor dyad, metacommunications regarding power and sex-role expectations may be conveyed to the counselees.

The syntactic context refers to the occurrence of a message relative to others in the communication matrix. For example, it is not uncommon for counselees to ask the same question two or more times during the course of the genetic counseling session. The meaning of a question such as, "What are our chances of having a normal child?" may be different when it is asked before the counselor has provided a risk estimate than when it comes afterwards. In one case the question may reflect a search for information, whereas in the other it may be a request for reassurance, even though the content of the message has remained the same.

Even though they may not be explicitly expressed, all messages contain requests (Satir, 1964). The requests may be for some specific action on the part of the receiver of the message. Most usually they are requests for sympathy, caring, or other feelings. Satir suggests that all messages contain requests for validation. Thus the simple statement, "The recurrence risk is one in four," may, and usually does, contain in its message, "Validate me and my ideas and knowledge by showing (through your responses) that you appreciate and understand me." Validation is often sought through circuitous routes and virtually every statement made either by the counselor or the counselees can be regarded as an attempt to obtain validation from each other. The major way counselors provide such validation is through their conveying to the counselees the feeling that they understand them.

The model of communication outlined above has several implications for genetic counseling. It underscores the concurrent interplay between content material and underlying psychological processes. It is not possible to convey a recurrence risk or other such information without simultaneously conveying multiple other messages. The latter include the counselors' own feelings about the genetic disorder, and their attitude toward the genetic risk as well as their perceptions of the counselees. For example, when a counselor says, "You have a three to one chance of having a normal baby," rather than "You have a one in four chance of having an affected baby," the metamessages in the two cases differ widely. For example, in the former case, the counselor may be conveying the metamessage, "I want you to like me and you will like me more if I do not talk about your chances of having an affected child." Or, perhaps the following: "I see you as fragile and incapable of handling the impact of a 'one in four' statement." The counselors' values may form part of the metamessage. For example, counselors may hold eugenics beliefs, and by conveying a risk figure emphasizing the possibility of an affected rather than a normal child, they may express the wish (consciously or not) that the counselees would not reproduce.

The model also suggests that by concentrating genetic counseling on a content level, the counselor probably conveys messages to the counselees that it is either unacceptable or risky to express their feelings; they run the risk of being misunderstood or emotionally rejected by the counselor. Such situations do not encourage the establishment of trust, and, without trust, counseling goals are not likely to be accomplished.

Because content and psychological issues are intermeshed in genetic counseling, the one-sided focus on one at the expense of the other is not likely to address counselees' needs. The content-oriented genetic counseling was inadequate because it did not encourage or allow the counselor to hear the metamessages underlying the questions posed by the counselees. Also, it prevented counselors from being aware of the metamessages that they were conveying to the counselees. In other words, the *process* of the counseling was tuned out. Similarly, genetic counseling without adequate attention to pertinent factual information is also likely to be ineffective as counselees need such facts to make informed decisions.

The model also addresses itself to the issue of team counseling in which content issues are handled by one professional, often a male, and emotional issues are entrusted to the care of someone else, not infrequently a female. This approach may convey multiple metamessages to the counselees regarding, for example, the relative values of rationality (high value) and emotions (low value). Also, it may suggest to the counselees that the counselor has a limited capacity to handle emotional issues.

Team approaches have psychological consequences. Philosophically, team approaches tend to emphasize a reason–emotion dualism [2] rather than an integrative synthesis of content and process issues; this may have an important influence on the counselees' experience of the counseling. The team approach may promote a further fragmentation of their experience that may, in turn, impede their ability to comprehend and integrate the information provided in the session. Moreover, the kind of team approach discussed above tends to recreate the traditional patriarchal family in which the father was the provider and the mother played a subordinate role. She often acted as an intermediary between the children and the feared father, who was emotionally distant and difficult to talk to.[3] The structure and role assignments in such families often had destructive consequences for the children as well as for the parents. As this model becomes increasingly unacceptable as a working structure for

[2] The conceptual split between reason and emotion is an old one in Western philosophy and probably reflects the fact that we have, in addition to a rational mode of consciousness, intuitive and other ways of knowing the world.

[3] In a recent article (Weiss, 1976), the role of the social worker in genetic counseling was pictured as benignly providing compensation for the counselor's emotional deficiencies and as acting as an intermediary between the latter and the counselees. I subscribe to the view that a system of counseling in which the actions of one component of the system threaten or reduce the self-esteem of the counselees and another part of the system supplies emotional "band-aids" cannot be as effective as one in which all components of the system are psychologically facilitative.

the contemporary family, its utility in the genetic counseling situation (or in medical practice in general) presumably will be called into question. Its application in the physician–nurse relationship is well known and its deleterious consequences on both patient care and on the "players" in the doctor–nurse game have been noted (Stein, 1967).

Effective Communication and Effective Counseling

In addition to the content of any particular genetic counseling session, the counselor communicates multiple other messages. The quality of these latter messages largely determines the degree to which the counselees have a sense of satisfaction, feel understood, and feel that their self-worth has been affirmed. In psychotherapy and in other areas of personal counseling, these factors constitute effective outcomes, as they are invariably associated with intellectual, cognitive, and affective growth. Considerable research suggests that the core factors needed to promote effective outcomes in psychotherapy and counseling are only a few in number (Truax & Carkhuff, 1966).

Carl Rogers and his students have suggested that the core dimensions which promote or inhibit effective counseling involve the provision, by the counselor, of messages containing adequate levels of empathy, respect or positive regard, genuineness, and concreteness.

Providing empathic understanding of another is considerably more than being sympathetic. In the latter, there is an emphasis on maintaining status and psychological boundaries between individuals whereas, in the former, some of these boundary lines are blurred so that the counselors allow themselves to "tune in" to the deeper levels of experience and feelings of the counselee, to experience and understand the latter's inner world and to communicate that understanding. Rogers (1957) writes that empathy consists of sensing "the client's private world as if it were your own, but without ever losing the 'as if' quality—this is empathy . . . [p. 99]." According to Carkhuff and Berenson (1967), at adequate levels of interpersonal functioning,

> the verbal or behavorial expressions of the . . . counselor . . . are essentially *interchangeable* with those of the [counselee] . . . in that they express essentially the same affect and meaning . . . [At optimum levels of interaction, the counselor's] responses . . . *add significantly* to the feelings and meanings of the [counselee] . . . in such a way as to express accurately feelings levels below what the person himself was able to express . . . [p. 5].

Positive regard refers to the counselor's ability to express respect, acceptance and caring for the counselee. Rogers (1957) writes that positive regard:

> means that there are no *conditions* of acceptance, no feeling of "I like you only *if* you are thus and so." It means a "prizing" of the person . . . [and] involves as much feeling of acceptance for the . . . expression of negative . . . feelings as for . . . "good" . . . feelings, as much acceptance of ways in which [the client] . . . is inconsistent as of ways in which he is consistent. It means a caring for the client, but not in a possessive way or in such a way as simply to satisfy the [counselor's] . . . own needs. It means a caring for the client as a *separate* person, with permission to have his own feelings, his own experiences [p. 98].

Positive regard is generally, but not always, communicated through warmth; it may also be communicated through anger ("I care for you enough to share my feelings of anger with you,").

Genuineness refers to the counselors' ability to be authentic and congruent with respect to what they say and what other cues convey that they are feeling. Optimally, genuineness means that the counselor "is freely and deeply himself, with his actual experience accurately represented by his awareness of himself. It is the opposite of presenting a facade, either knowingly or unknowingly [Rogers, 1957, p. 97]."

Concreteness "involves the fluent, direct, and complete expression of specific feelings and experiences, regardless of their emotional content . . . [Carkhuff & Berenson, 1967, p. 29]." At minimally facilitative levels of interaction, the counselor enables the counselee to discuss personally relevant material in specific and concrete terms rather than in terms of vagaries and abstractions. Optimally the counselor "is *always* helpful in guiding discussion so that the [counselee] . . . may discuss fluently, directly and completely specific feelings and experiences [Carkhuff & Berenson, 1967, p. 7]."

Considerable data suggest that all counseling interactions may have positive or negative, constructive or deteriorative consequences for the counselees. Measured on a variety of indices, effective counseling has been shown to occur when the counselor provides high levels of empathy, positive regard, genuineness, and concreteness. Conversely, deteriorative consequences occur when low levels of these dimensions are provided (Carkhuff & Berenson, 1967).

One of the elementary, nonetheless important, messages which emerges from the work of a variety of clinicians is that the issue of effective communication is not unique to the counseling encounter. It is present in all human interactions. Another way of stating it is that the dimensions of human behavior which lead to effective communication in everyday life are the very same as those which lead to positive counseling outcomes. This implies that the techniques by which genetic counselors might improve their counseling skills and possibly make the counseling process more effective do not reside in any set of mysteries. They are available in the interaction skills most of us already possess. Like most skills, these abilities become more effective with training and practice.

Decision Making

Helping counselees reach appropriate reproductive decisions is an important aspect of genetic counseling. How and why couples make the decisions they do following genetic counseling is poorly understood. Recent findings on how persons weigh information and judge uncertain situations may have a bearing on the decision-making process in genetic counseling. This research may be summarized as follows: First, it has been found that the interpretation of statistical probability is highly subjective (Pearn, 1973). For example, a risk figure of one in four may mean one thing for a person one day in an optimistic frame of mind and another when in a pessimistic state.[4] Also, even though they may behave as if a genetic risk figure means the same thing to each, it probably has different meanings for the counselor and counselees.

Second, in the face of uncertainty, thinking is directed toward simplifying the assessment of probabilities and predicted outcomes of various choices (Tversky & Kahneman, 1974). The processes of simplification may involve the use of heuristic principles (e.g., anchoring and adjustment) which may lead to biased assessments and hence to possible major errors of judgment. For example, prior to counseling, a counselee may have a preconceived idea of a recurrence risk which may serve as an anchor or starting point that is adjusted either upward or downward as a result of counseling. Thus, one counselee may have expected a risk of 100% and may be overjoyed that the actual risk is "as low as" 50%. Another person may have expected a risk of only 1% and may be "stunned" by a risk of 5%. In the first case, a relatively high risk may be minimized unrealistically whereas in the second case, a relatively low genetic risk may be unrealistically magnified relative to their respective anchoring points.

Third, individuals with a knowledge of statistics may be as prone to

[4] The optimist–pessimist dimension is sometimes used to describe personality differences in the genetic counseling literature. This dimension might better be thought of as situation-specific, transient attitudinal variations. Personality encompasses relatively stable and enduring behavioral and psychological qualities of the individual.

errors of judgment in evaluating some uncertain continqencies as are laypersons (Kahneman & Tversky, 1973). Thus, relatively greater intellect or education may not necessarily lead to greater understanding when the matter at hand has some emotional relevance for the person.

Lastly, it appears that the sources of judgmental bias may have a cognitive basis. Slovic (1972) suggests that the biases have a persistent quality not unlike that of perceptual illusions. Thus, human rationality may have bounds, imposed by cognitive mechanisms, which make it difficult to use genetic risk information to optimal rational advantage in reproductive decisions. These findings are consistent with the observations of psychoanalysts and other clinicians who have worked with persons in the throes of making important life decisions. It is repeatedly noted that nonrational factors play a major role in reaching such decisions. Rational decision making in genetic counseling is an ideal. Providing information to promote rational decisions may be successfully accomplished, yet decisions may appear to be capricious or unexpected (in the eyes of the counselor). This occurs because rational thinking is applied relative to one's cognitive schemas or inner models of reality rather than to external reality. It is likely that the respective cognitive schemas of geneticists and of counselees may be significantly different. Thus, in the world-view of the counselees they may be behaving rationally and in their own self-interest, but from the counselor's point of view, they may be failing to act responsibly or rationally. In Chapter 5, the specific pragmatics of facilitating the autonomous decision making of the counselees will be examined in greater detail.

Coping Processes

Out of the literature on grief reactions (Lindemann, 1944), ego and cognitive psychology, and other lines of psychological–psychiatric thinking, evidence has been marshalled concerning the coping responses of nonpsychiatric populations to major life stresses (Murphy, 1960; Kroeber, 1963; Haan, 1963; Chodoff, Friedman, & Hamburg, 1964; Lazarus, 1966; Coelho, Hamburg, & Adams, 1974; Horowitz, 1976). This literature has a special relevance for genetic counseling. It has become increasingly evident that the content material of genetic counseling, the diagnosis or occurrence of a genetic disorder and the threat of its occurrence are often perceived as major stresses. Like other stresses, they require internal processing, working-through, and, often, the acquisition of novel behavioral responses. Life stresses such as genetic disorders are opportunities, albeit sometimes painful ones, to which the individual may respond in ways that produce important affective, cognitive, and intellectual changes. For this reason there is a fine line between what the counselor might accomplish in genetic counseling and that accomplished by the counselor in psychotherapy. During periods of stress, one is particularly vulnerable and thus tends to magnify the effects of professional interventions. Genetic counselors need to understand that their interventions may have major ramifications for the counselees that go far beyond the borders of the counseling session itself.

Studies of individuals facing important life stresses and transitions indicate that, in general, there are three major stages of coping with such phenomena. At first there is a response of protest or a resistance to accept that one's world has changed. As the impact of the stress sinks in, a period of disorganization occurs in which the person's inner sense of the world begins to alter. Lastly, a period of reorganization ensues in which the individual develops a new way of looking at the world and, often, new ways of behaving.

The major stages of coping with stress-evoking events may be divided into the following phases.[5]

INITIAL REALIZATION OR OUTCRY

This phase is usually accompanied by intense distress.

DENIAL

Denial is often accompanied by a sense of numbness. At first, little affect may be expressed, feelings might be blocked out or denied, the event may be disbelieved, painful thoughts including reminders of the event may be inhibited and pleasant ones may be evoked. As this phase continues an increase of affect may be exhibited. In these initial stages, weeping may serve both as a protest and as an attempt, on the level of magical thinking, of bringing the lost object back again (Wolff, 1977).

INTRUSION

Thoughts about the event or lost object may break through into consciousness. The person may exhibit a yearning for or preoccupation with thoughts of the lost object or the stress event accompanied with feelings

[5] Several excellent accounts of coping have been published (e.g., Hamburg & Adams, 1967; Lazarus, Averill & Opton, 1974). Others have labelled the various stages of coping differently than the one used here. I follow the schema advanced by Horowitz (1976). His views are attractive because they synthesize findings from several sources (psychodynamic as well as cognitive psychology) from the viewpoint of the clinician.

of profound sadness or depression.[6] This phase is marked by an oscillation between periods of intense feeling and periods of conscious or unconscious avoidance of feelings and of repression. Anger may be expressed toward physicians and paramedical personnel as well as toward family members and other "reminders" of health or of the lost object.

The repeated recurrence of thoughts and memories of the stress event serves an important adaptational function in that at each recurrence the individual is, so-to-speak, given another chance to relive, reexperience, and reappraise the original event. In so doing, a desensitization occurs; that is, the original event gradually loses its "sting." With each successive recurrence, the memory begins to lose its intrusive and involuntary nature and may be revised both in content and in form. These changes suggest that a progressive mastery of the experience has occurred.

In the denial and intrusive subphases, the individual's thoughts and affects tend to be organized around certain commonly appearing themes:

(*a*) *A fear of repetition.* If it happened once, it could happen again. For many genetic diseases, this fear may have a realistic basis. The thought of repetition may be as feared as much as the event itself.

(*b*) *Shame over helplessness.* Stressful situations, such as the diagnosis of a genetic disorder, attack the unrealistic, nevertheless ubiquitous, belief that one has total control over one's life. The loss of control imposed by the occurrence of genetic disorders is often experienced with shame.

(*c*) *Rage and fault-finding.* The need to know, "Why has this happened to me?" and to assign blame often leads to anger at anyone who might be at fault, rationally or not. This may include the affected child, one's spouse (especially in X-linked disorders), the physician and others. The rage may evoke destructive fantasies that may, in turn, conflict with one's sense of conscience, leading to further feelings of guilt or shame. Destructive fantasies may also trigger fears of losing control and impulsively acting out the fantasy.

(*d*) *Survivor guilt.* This has been described among survivors of concentration camps and of other traumatic situations. It is also seen among the unaffected siblings of persons with genetic disorders The guilt may have two sources, the belief that one has eluded fate at the expense of

---

[6] The genetic counselor needs to be alert to differentiate between the sadness due to grief and that due to depression. In the former, the world appears bleak, empty, and meaningless whereas in the latter, the persons experience themselves as empty and worthless; that is they appear to be more preoccupied with themselves than with the lost object. In the grieving person, self-esteem remains intact (Peretz, 1970; Wolff, 1977).

the victim and the belief that one is selfish because one wishes to be a survivor.

(*e*) *Fear of identification with affected individuals.* In early childhood, persons are not cognitively conceptualized as being discretely separate from one's self. Stress may evoke thoughts that if another has been harmed by a genetic disorder, then one may or will be harmed oneself. One may then begin to think of oneself as actually a victim even though no correspondence exists with reality.

(*f*) *Sadness over loss, real or symbolic, of persons, external resources, and aspects of the self, including one's self esteem.*

Research summarized by Horowitz (1976) suggests that the problems outlined above frequently provide the ideational and emotional contents which tend to be warded off during initial stages of coping with stress. Also, they comprise the developmental themes around which current and past responses to stress tend to interdigitate. Because of this, it is often difficult to tease out the extent to which responses to genetic disorders or other stress events are due to recent life events or to past developmental problems and unresolved conflicts.

WORKING THROUGH

This phase consists of repeated cycles of denial and intrusion, in which the intensity of emotions diminishes and the cyclicity loses its peremptory quality. There is a beginning of an acceptance of the reality of the original stress event. A turning point appears to be reached in which there appears to be an abandonment of old modes of behavior and thought.

COMPLETION

Completion involves the termination of internalized states of stress via cognitive processing. The person may become active in terminating the stress state either by overt changes of usual behavior or, as in the case of the dying person, actively becoming passive (e.g., separating oneself from one's survivors prior to death) (Kubler-Ross, 1969). In real life, completion seldom occurs and the person frequently reexperiences waves of grief and oscillations between denial–numbness and intrusion–repetitions. However, the frequency and intensity tend to diminish as well as their autonomous nature. Recollections of the original stress become increasingly dependent on the presence of associational triggers to memories of loss.

The five phases just enumerated represent the general response tendencies noted by many clinicians in their investigations of different stress states. Individual differences have been seen in the sequence at which the first three phases are entered and in the frequency with which the various phases may be repeated. Personality styles may influence the responses to the various subphases and to the counselor's interventions. Also, stress events generally activate a complex set of associational responses, some portions of which may be more conflicted or difficult to accept than others. Thus, at any given time in the coping sequence, one set of ideational and affective responses may be in one phase and another set may be in a functionally different phase (Horowitz, 1976). This suggests that the arguments usually advanced in the literature about not providing genetic counseling during early stages of the coping process are open to question. Such arguments may be rationalizations for avoiding the anticipated emotional intensity of the counselees. The fact is, *emphatic genetic counseling may be provided at any point of the coping process.* It is ironic that the point at which the counselees require contact, emotional support, and help in understanding their inner experience appears to be the very time when helping professionals, not infrequently including mental health persons, are least likely to want to be involved with them. If their self-worth has been damaged by the diagnosis of a genetic disorder and/or if they are feeling guilt and shame, the professional's attitude may confirm that they are not worthy of being helped and that the fantasies of why they should be guilty and ashamed are correct.

Genetic counselors can play an important role in helping the counselees cope with the diagnosis or occurrence of a genetic disorder. As resource persons, they may serve as an important source of information regarding the particular genetic disorder, its management, course, possible problems and burdens, and so forth. They may also provide information regarding pertinent community agencies and/or parent support groups. Counselees need this information in order to separate fact from fantasy and to make relevant decisions. By imparting information empathically, that is, tuning-in to the counselees' needs and providing the most relevant and adequate information—neither too much nor too little—counselors convey the message that they understand, care, and are "there" for them. This is particularly important for couples with little or no external social support system.

Genetic counselors can also help the counselees deal with their feelings and keep their affect from overwhelming and disorganizing their efforts to make decisions or take reality-based actions. The counselors can help them separate past associations and anticipated difficulties from the here-

and-now issues with which they need to deal. Also, they can (and should) legitimize the counselees' feelings by conveying the message that they are entitled to feel what they are feeling, whatever it is, sadness, anger, guilt, etc. and thus confirm the appropriateness of their behavior and their worth as human beings. The experience of being accepted by another person goes a long way to ease the pain one is feeling and to restore one's self-esteem.

Lastly, the counselors can prepare the counselees for problems or difficulties they might not have anticipated (e.g., abortion in the case of preamniocentesis counseling). Considerable data suggest that when people anticipate or are aware of an impending crisis or stress, it assists them to do anticipatory grief work (Lindemann, 1944), to start working through their feelings and to make plans to cope adequately with the stress (Lazarus *et al.*, 1974; Janis & Mann, 1976).

Like any other professional intervention, genetic counseling may be used to help persons experiencing grief or dealing with crisis to resume previous levels of functioning (homeostasis approach) or it may be used as a means of achieving more effective and differentiated modes of functioning (growth model). The goals, values, and attitudes of the counselors may play a crucial role in this regard, because their interventions may convey differential expectations of the potentiality for growth. If the counselors believe that the cognitive, intellectual, and affective growth of the counselees is a possible and desirable end of genetic counseling, their interventions may be qualitatively different from those of counselors who do not share that belief.

References

Bateson, G., Jackson, D. D., Haley, J. & Weakland, J. Toward a theory of schizophrenia. *Behavioral Science*, 1956, *1*, 251–264.

Carkhuff, R. R. & Berenson, B. G. *Beyond counseling and psychotherapy*. New York: Holt, Rinehart and Winston, 1967.

Chodoff, P., Friedman, S. B. & Hamburg, D. A. Stress, defenses and coping behavior: Observations in parents of children with malignant disease. *American Journal of Psychiatry*, 1964, *120*, 743–749.

Coelho, G. V., Hamburg, D. A. & Adams, J. E. *Coping and adaptation*. New York: Basic Books, 1974.

Gillum, R. F. & Borsky, A. J. Diagnosis and management of patient noncompliance. *Journal of the American Medical Association*, 1974, *228*, 1563–1567.

Haan, N. Proposed model of ego functioning: Coping and defense mechanisms in relationship to IQ change. *Psychological Monographs*, 1963, *77*(8), 1–23.

Haley, J. *Strategies of psychotherapy*. New York: Grune and Stratton, 1963.

Hamburg, D. A. & Adams, J. E. A perspective on coping behavior. *Archives of General Psychiatry*, 1967, *17*, 277–284.

Horowitz, M. J. *Stress response syndromes*. New York: Jason Aronson, 1976.

Janis, I. L. & Mann, L. Coping with decisional conflict. *American Scientist*, 1976, *64*, 657–667.

Kahneman, D. & Tversky, A. On the psychology of prediction. *Psychological Review*, 1973, *80*, 237–251.

Korsch, B. M. & Negrete, V. F. Doctor-patient communication. *Scientific American*, 1972, *227*, 66–74.

Kroeber, T. The coping functions of the ego mechanisms. In R. White (Ed.), *The study of lives*. New York: Atherton Press, 1963.

Kubler-Ross, E. *On death and dying*. New York: Macmillan and Co., 1969.

Lazarus, R. S. *Psychological stress and the coping process*. New York: McGraw-Hill, 1966.

Lazarus, R. S., Averill, J. R. & Opton, Jr., E. M. The psychology of coping: Issues of research and assessment. In G. V. Coelho, D. A. Hamburg & J. E. Adams (Eds.), *Coping and adaptation*. New York: Basic Books, 1974.

Leonard, C. O., Chase, G. & Childs, B. Genetic counseling: A consumer's view. *New England Journal of Medicine*, 1972, *287*, 433–439.

Lindemann, E. Symptomatology and management of acute grief. *American Journal of Psychiatry*, 1944, *101*, 141–148.

Murphy, L. B. Coping devices and defense mechanisms in relation to autonomous ego functions. *Menninger Clinic Bulletin*, 1960, *24*, 144–153.

Pearn, J. H. Patients' subjective interpretation of risks offered in genetic counseling. *Journal of Medical Genetics*, 1973, *10*, 129–134.

Peretz, D. Reaction to loss. In B. Schoenberg, A. C. Carr, D. Peretz & A. H. Kutscher (Eds.), *Loss and grief: Psychological management in medical practice*. New York: Columbia Univ. Press, 1970.

Rogers, C. R. The necessary and sufficient conditions of therapeutic personality change. *Journal of Consulting Psychology*, 1957, *21*, 95–103.

Ruesch, J. & Bateson, G. *Communication: The social matrix of psychiatry*. New York: W. W. Norton and Co., 1951.

Satir, V. *Conjoint family therapy*. Palo Alto: Science and Behavior Books, 1964.

Slovic, P. From Shakespeare to Simon: Speculations—and some evidence—about man's ability to process information. *Oregon Research Institute Research Monograph*, 1972, *12*, 1–29.

Sorenson, J. R. Sociological and psychological factors in applied human genetics. In B. Hilton, D. Callahan, M. Harris, P. Condliffe & B. Berkley (Eds.), *Ethical issues in human genetics*. New York: Plenum Press, 1973.

Sorenson, J. R. Genetic counseling: Some psychological considerations. In M. Lipkin, Jr. and P. T. Rowley (Eds.), *Genetic responsibility*. New York: Plenum Press, 1974.

Stein, L. I. The doctor–nurse game. *Archives of General Psychiatry*, 1967, *16*, 699–703.

Truax, C. B. & Carkhuff, R. R. *Introduction to counseling and psychotherapy: Training and practice*. Chicago: Aldine Press, 1966.

Tversky, A. & Kahneman, D. Judgment under uncertainty: Heuristics and biases. *Science*, 1974, *185*, 1124–1131.

Watzlawick, P., Beavin, J. H. & Jackson, D. D. *Pragmatics of human communication*. Palo Alto: Science and Behavior Books, 1967.

Weiss, J. O. Social work and genetic counseling. *Social Work in Health Care*, 1976, *2*, 5–12.

Wolff, C. T. Loss, grief, and mourning in adults. In R. C. Simons and H. Pardes (Eds.), *Understanding human behavior in health and illness*. Baltimore: Williams and Wilkins Co., 1977.

The Counselor–Counselee Relationship

4

Seymour Kessler

At the heart of the genetic counseling encounter is the counselor–counselee relationship. No discussion of genetic counseling would be complete without a consideration of the meaning and implications of this relationship. The need to do so is underscored by evidence (Goldstein & Dean, 1966; Truax & Carkhuff, 1966) strongly suggesting that the nature of the relationship in a counseling situation, in itself, is the most important determinant of counseling outcomes. Patterson (1966) suggests that much of what counselors do or provide in the way of content may be "superfluous or unrelated to their effectiveness; in fact, it is likely that much of their success . . . occurs in spite of what they do . . . [p. 504]." If this is true in genetic counseling, it has broad implications for the delivery of genetic disease services and for the training of providers of genetic counseling.

Models of Counselor–Counselee Relationships

Sorenson (1973, 1974) has taken the lead in exploring the counselor–counselee relationship in genetic counseling. As a sociologist, he places major emphasis on the respective social roles of the participants in the counseling and on the role negotiations which occur around two major issues: (*a*) the kind of information provided by the counselor and (*b*) the counselor's perceived role as a decision maker. He describes several models of interaction ranging, on one side, from the counselor offering

53

GENETIC COUNSELING
Psychological Dimensions

direct advice or prescribing the actions the counselees should take to one in which the counselor simply provides factual information and neither assists the counselees to interpret the information nor provides them with advice on what decisions to make. The former case describes the traditional physician–patient relationship whereas in the latter, the counselor attempts to establish a teacher–student[1] relationship (Sorenson, 1974).

The sociological analysis of the counselor–counselee relationship provides a limited perspective on the nature of this interaction. For example, in terms of the social roles involved, the two models described above appear to be vastly different. Psychologically, however, the two models may be seen as variations on the same theme. Both incorporate elements of the parent–child interaction; the counselor is the powerful, knowing parent and the counselee is the helpless, dependent child. Thus, in both models the power-dependency differential between counselor and counselee is the same. In the physician–patient model, the parent is an authoritarian one whereas in the teacher–student model, the parent is permissive and expects that the child will behave in a mature, responsible, adult way even though he or she is treated like a child. In one case, the parent exercises too much power whereas in the other, the parent fails to invest the child with any of the power. Thus, both models of counseling have the same end result, that is, they tend to render the counselees powerless and make it difficult for them to assert their autonomy with respect to the decisions they might need to make.

A better understanding of both the sociological and psychological nature of the counselor–counselee relationship in genetic counseling would be most desirable, particularly if this relationship is to be used to maximum effectiveness. The psychological analyses currently available concern the physician–patient relationship (Szasz & Hollender, 1956). However, by extrapolation, these models may be extended to include all relationships between helping professionals and the patients, clients, counselees, and so on, with whom they interact. Szasz and Hollender discuss three types of relationships. One type is organized in an *activity–passivity* frame of reference. The professional actively does something to the client, whereas the latter is inert or unable to respond. This relationship occurs in the physician's treatment of a patient in coma. On a psychological level, it is a recreation of the parent–infant relationship.

A second approach involves a *guidance–cooperation* model. Here the

---

[1] As a model of teacher–student interaction, this approach is hardly adequate. A teacher who did not explore the implications of his or her subject matter and who did not place the teachings in a historical, philosophical, psychological, or other perspective would be a total bore!

professional tells the client what to do and the latter expects the professional to do so. This describes the traditional physician–patient interaction, the prototype of which is the parent–child relationship. The physician–parent is acknowledged as having greater wisdom and power and the patient–child's role is to show respect and to obey. This paradigm is often applied in the treatment of acute medical disorders.

Lastly, Szasz and Hollender describe a model of *mutual participation* in which the professional strives to help the clients help themselves. This type of relationship is generally needed in the treatment of chronic illnesses and in many psychotherapeutic encounters. It approximates adult–adult interactions.

In the genetic counseling interaction, aspects of both the *guidance–cooperation* and *mutual participation* models are found. Thus, these models will be examined in greater detail.

The guidance–cooperation model has been developed most succinctly by the sociologist Talcott Parsons and, more recently, by Siegler and Osmond (1974). Parsons (1951) stresses the complementary nature of the physician–patient relationship. Each participant has a social role to play around the issue of health care; there is a mutuality of expectations and socially prescribed ways of acting. The patient enters the sick role. The physicians use their Aesculapian authority (Siegler & Osmond, 1974) and prestige to confer this role and to heal the patient. In the sick role, the patient is not held responsible for the illness, and is exempted from some or all social obligations. According to Parsons, it is the obligation of the sick person to seek medical help and to cooperate with the physician in the treatment.

In genetic counseling, interactions in which the counselors use their authority as a means of altering the counselees' behavior are in line with the guidance-cooperation model. The authority may be exerted consciously or unconsciously. For example, when the counselors provide advice (e.g., "If I were in your position, I would do such and such."), they are consciously attempting to influence counselee behavior within the framework of the guidance–cooperation model. Unconscious uses of one's authority may follow multiple different pathways, some of which have been discussed earlier in Chapter 3. The possibility of unconsciously influencing counselee behavior has been acknowledged by several geneticists. Fraser (1974) suggests that the genetic counselor needs to "avoid projecting his own personality defects into the situation . . . [p. 650]", and others have warned against putting one's own "hang-ups" on the counselees. This may be easier said than done as, most usually, we are not aware of our own personality quirks, have little understanding of their dynamics and, as a consequence, have little control over how they are used and how they impact others.[2]

Whereas in the guidance–cooperation approach both participants assume asymmetry in their relationship and agree that the physician or counselor knows "best," the mutual participation model assumes a symmetrical relationship and the physician–counselor does not profess to know what is best for the patient–counselee. It is the mutual search for this that is the essence of their relationship. Describing the main aspects of this model, Szasz and Hollender write:

> This model is predicated on the postulate that equality among human beings is desirable. . . . Psychologically, mutuality rests on complex processes of identification—which facilitate conceiving of others in terms of oneself—together with maintaining and tolerating the discrete individuality of the observer and the observed.[3] It is crucial to this type of interaction that the participants (1) have approximately equal power, (2) be mutually interdependent . . . , and (3) engage in activity that will be in some ways satisfying to both [p. 587].

Szasz and Hollender realize that this model represents a marked departure from the traditional conceptualization of the physician–patient relationship. They write:

> The model of mutual participation . . . is essentially foreign to medicine. This relationship, characterized by a high degree of empathy, has elements often associated with the notions of friendship and partnership and the imparting of expert advice. The physician may be said to help the patient to help himself. The physician's gratification cannot stem from power or from the control over someone else. His satisfactions are derived from more abstract kinds of mastery, which are as yet poorly understood [p. 588].

Despite its unfamiliarity, the mutual participation model has much to commend it for the purposes of genetic counseling. In many cases, we do not know what the best course of action might be for a given couple. Even in the case where a couple is faced with the decision of aborting or not aborting a fetus with a definitely diagnosed life-debilitating genetic disease, it is by no means clear what their "best" decision should be, in terms of their moral, ethical, psychological, and practical needs.

The guidance–cooperation model assumes that the professionals are

---

[2] Psychotherapy often deals with this very problem. Although virtually no geneticist has urged that one of the essentials in the training of genetic counselors ought to be an intensive experience in personal psychotherapy, it is clear that such an experience would be highly desirable.

[3] Compare this statement with Roger's definition of empathy (p. 42)—Ed.

experts—and they are. The physicians, for example, are experts in the domain of diagnosis and treatment. However, outside this arena, they increasingly lose the status of an expert, and when it comes to the application of genetic technology and to the dilemmas and choices it poses for the individual and for society, the physician and geneticist may be no more expert than the philosopher, sociologist, psychologist, minister, or other nonphysician professionals.

Furthermore, the value of nondirectiveness in counseling may be more compatible with a model of mutual participation than with the more traditional model. By relating to the counselees as parents, the counselors imply that they will take responsibility for their decision. Relating to them on the level of one adult to another allows the onus of responsibility to rest (where it should) with the counselees and conveys a message of trust that the latter are capable of making decisions for themselves.

Perhaps the most cogent reason for moving toward a model of mutual participation is that the traditional model of physician–patient interaction, like other relationships based on a power differential, often is a self-defeating one. For example, consider the issue of patient noncompliance, "one of the major unsolved therapeutic problems confronting the medical profession today [Gillum & Borsky, 1974]." Davis (1968) and others suggest that a third or more of patients do not comply with their physician's advice or prescriptions. Psychological, social, and environmental factors, the specific therapeutic regimen involved, and the quality and nature of the physician–patient interaction are all believed to be involved in fostering noncompliant behavior. Physicians generally deal with noncompliance by denying the magnitude of the problem or through attempts to persuade the patient by giving explanations of expected behavior, rational arguments, threats, and, finally, by withdrawing their services.[4] None of these responses appear to be effective in changing the patient's noncompliant behavior (Gillum & Borsky, 1974), and the physician often ends up feeling frustrated and angry. To add insult to injury, nonphysician health personnel and some lay persons often blame the physicians for creating, through their own behavior, the problem of noncompliance in the first place. In turn the physician tends to accuse the patient for being uncooperative and obstructionistic.

Family therapists will readily recognize the similarity of the scenario of the noncompliant patient to that of the deliquent, acting-out child in the traditionally patriarchal family. Like the former, the child is generally labeled as antagonistic and rebellious and identified as the patient

[4] This latter tactic is an expression of the physician's frustration with the patient. It symbolizes the parent's punitive withdrawal of affection and attention from the "misbehaving" child.

needing treatment ("If only he or she would behave, everything in the family would be O.K."). Therapeutic work with such family systems frequently reveals that the distribution of power in the system is asymmetrical—there are haves and have nots—and there are implicit myths governing the behavior of the members of the system, namely that power is finite and that there just isn't enough to go around. Such systems generally also have a rule of conduct which disallows comments on the asymmetrical distribution of power; anyone, including the therapist, who breaks this rule is subject to attack and ostracism. It is often found that the acting-out behavior of the identified patient is a means of dealing with the inner sense of powerlessness in which the behavior becomes a vehicle for influencing one's environment and maintaining one's integrity and autonomy even at the expense of punishment and, sometimes, self-injury. This may also account for the behavior of the noncompliant patient.

The fact that the physician may sometimes become the ultimate "victim" of the traditional physician–patient relationship is insufficiently attended to in the medical literature. Difficulties in obtaining appropriate health care for themselves and their families (Bowden & Burstein, 1974), marital dysfunctions (Evans, 1965; Vaillant, Sobowak & McArthur, 1972; Krell & Miles, 1976), a high incidence of suicide (a'Brook, Hailstone & McLauchlan, 1967), and other human problems may be the personal price paid by some practitioners to maintain the system of omnipotence of the traditional physician–patient relationship.

For several reasons, then, the adoption of a model of mutual participation would be a desirable step in genetic counseling. The absence of absolute standards of right and wrong, limitations of counselor expertise with respect to other persons' reproductive and health decisions, the greater compatibility with the value of nondirectiveness, and the possible negative consequences for professional and client alike of a system based on a power differential all argue for the abandonment or modification of the traditional physician–patient relationship as a standard model for providing genetic counseling. Furthermore, contemporary trends toward the greater expression of patients' rights and greater involvement in their own health care are, presumably, more compatible with a model of counseling which maximizes counselee autonomy than one which vests responsibility and decision-making powers in the professional.

It is conceivable that some genetic counselors may have difficulty relating to either the guidance–cooperation or the mutual participation models, both seeming too extreme for their needs or tastes. It is likely that many such professionals already incorporate aspects of both models into their counseling. This would be expected of a field undergoing flux and in a situation in which the customary role relationships are not totally applicable. The consequences of using a mixed model will need to be explored and monitored. On one hand, a mixed model may be a reasonable compromise from both the professional's viewpoint and that of the counselees, as it would allow each participant in the encounter to adjust to the novel demand aspects of genetic counseling. On the other hand, counselees may experience the inconsistent aspects of the model and may view the counselor much like an unpredictable parent, demanding child-like behavior at one moment and adult behavior the next. Under such conditions, communication between the counselor and counselee is likely to be incongruent. Interprofessional relationships are also likely to be inconsistent and, possibly, filled with conflict, mostly of a covert nature. For example, each move toward autonomy on the part of nonphysician professionals may be viewed as a challenge or threat on the part of physician practitioners and thus strongly resisted. Genetic counseling teams, consisting of physician and nonphysician professionals, may become extensions of the mixed attitudes of the parent–child and adult–adult models. Relationships between counselors and counselees may be along adult–adult lines, but, within the team itself, a distinct pecking order may develop along parent–child lines. Hopefully, such situations will be seen as transitional steps to a reorganization of genetic disease services along greater person-oriented rather than technologically oriented lines.

Genetic Counseling and Behavior Control

All forms of counseling have the potential of influencing behavior. In fact, an argument can be made that some influence *must* occur if counseling is to be effective. One of the implicit understandings of genetic counseling is that some aspects of the counselees' attitudes, beliefs, and behavior regarding a genetic disease and/or its sequelae will be modified as a function of the counseling. A motive-less request for information or a motive-less imparting of it is an unrealistic paradigm of genetic counseling. Persons desire personally relevant information, and counselors provide such information for many conscious and unconscious reasons. For example, models of health behavior generally postulate that a perceived susceptibility or risk is one of the important factors which motivates individuals to seek professional counsel (Maiman & Becker, 1974).

Once counselees receive personally relevant information, it is doubtful that their inner worlds would remain untouched or unchanged. Ambivalences may be intensified or resolved, feelings about the self modified, one's understanding about the past or future altered and interpersonal relations changed. Whether we wish it or not, genetic counselors, like counselors in other areas, are agents of behavior change.

In recent years, geneticists have become increasingly involved in activities which have broad implications in terms of human behavior and its control. These include the development of pertinent educational programs in the elementary and secondary schools and colleges, and of other public education programs designed to inform people about the nature and impact of genetic disease. Such educational efforts are often associated with large-scale screening programs and aim to alert the public to such genetic disorders as sickle-cell disease and Tay-Sachs disease, and to motivate persons to come for testing, generally to detect heterozygote individuals who would be at especially high risk for having affected children. These programs have obvious public health benefits and are often funded by governmental agencies because of their cost-effectiveness with respect to avoiding expensive medical treatment, years of possible institutionalization, as well as enormous personal and family tragedy. Nevertheless, these programs carry the potential of behavior control and a concomitant danger to human freedom.

It needs to be recognized that a sophisticated technology already exists to manipulate and control human behavior (London, 1969). If behavior control technology can be used to motivate individuals and groups to purchase particular products, to vote for one candidate over another or to rally support for a war, it can also be used to motivate masses of people to subject themselves to genetic disease detection procedures or to modify their marriage or reproductive choices. London (1969) discusses the dangers inherent in even the most benevolent of behavioral control programs. He writes:

> The danger to a free society from behavior technology . . . is not that a few tyrannical rogues will first propagandize us into giving them power and then scramble our brains or our television sets to keep it. The danger is that even its most benevolent use runs the risk of eroding freedom when it take place *by the decision of anyone other than the person on whom it is used* . . . The ethical challenge emphasized by behavior technology is that of how to preserve or enhance individual liberty under circumstances where its suppression will frequently be justified not only by the common welfare but for the individual's happiness [p. 208].

London's caveat is particularly pertinent in the social application of genetic technology (Taviss, 1971). The dilemma frequently encountered in the delivery of genetic disease services is that any attempt to educate must have an intended goal in mind and this goal invariably involves an attempt to persuade or to guide human actions in a way consistent with the educator's value system. In addition, informed permission of the target individual or group cannot be obtained without engaging in an attempt to persuade such persons to give the permission. How then are genetic services to be provided with full informed consent and, at the same time, with a full concern for the rights of the individual? Somewhere in the course of this health-care delivery process, an interaction between the consumer-counselee and a trained ally must occur, whose ultimate goal hopefully will be to preserve or enhance the former's autonomy and freedom. Herein, lies a major raison d'être of genetic counseling.

The counselor–counselee relationship in genetic counseling is an important vehicle by which the individuals' freedom to choose their own life direction might either be sustained or eroded. From the counselors' end of things, the degree to which they are commited to two interrelated beliefs may contribute to the ultimate outcome in this regard. These are: (a) the belief that individuals' rights should receive priority over those of society or agencies of society and (b) the belief that individuals are capable and desirous of managing their own life affairs.

An allegiance to the primacy of the individual is but one of several value orientations espoused by practitioners of genetic counseling (Lappé, 1973). One's values may not only influence the counselor's behavior and interventions in the genetic counseling encounter, but may also have important social policymaking implications. The latter may include decisions influencing the extent to which health services and therapies are made available to affected persons and the degree to which the development of new therapeutic procedures is encouraged. Lappé suggests that the values of genetic counselors may largely reflect the orientations of the medical subspecialties or disciplines from which the counselor comes.

Although many geneticists have expressed their commitment to individual prerogatives, many also hold additional values which may compete with their allegiance to individual primacy. For many geneticists, an allegiance to the individual is (or may come to be) in conflict with a strong desire to prevent disease, minimize human suffering, protect the human gene pool, and other worthy goals. Also, for some, the "bottom-line" faith or confidence in the individual and his or her striving for competence and mastery (White, 1972) has either never been established or has not been strengthened by one's experiences or academic and professional training. For these practitioners, it is understandable why they might be attracted to or motivated by allegiances other than one to individual primacy.

In the face of conflicting values, it may be difficult to champion individual prerogatives without the sustaining personal belief that individuals have the capacity and desire to direct their own existence and destiny.

At least two issues need to be taken into account in assisting genetic counselors to be effective agents of the individual and helping them maintain a consistent ideological commitment to individual autonomy. First, it should be recognized that the needs of research and of service may sometimes come into conflict. The two enterprises are often intertwined in the delivery of genetic disease services and sometimes do not adequately account for the human elements introduced by the fact that the practitioner and biomedical scientist may have different world views with respect to their basic ways of conceptualizing problems, their patterns of reasoning, modes of action, and the criteria they use in making judgments (Kennedy, 1973). The increasing participation of genetic associates in the genetic counseling process may provide a major means of balancing or avoiding the conflicts raised by research and service needs of many medical centers.

Second, genetic counselors need to be encouraged to obtain the depth of self-knowledge and the requisite counseling skills to allow them to guide the counselees through the shoals of the various conflicts introduced by the differing perceptions, needs, and values of individuals, institutions, and society such that individual freedom and prerogative is maintained or enhanced. In this regard, a thorough preparation in the principles and practices of counseling as they relate to the psychosocial issues of genetic disease, bioethical dilemmas, and human growth should be the central focus of training and education of genetic counselors in addition to training in genetics.

References

Bowden, C. L. & Burstein, A. G. *Psychosocial bases of medical practice*. Baltimore: Williams and Wilkins Co., 1974.

a'Brook, M. F., Hailstone, J. D. & McLauchlan, I. E. J. Psychiatric illness in the medical profession. *British Journal of Psychiatry*, 1967, *113*, 1013–1023.

Davis, M. S. Variations in patients' compliance with doctors' advice: An empirical analysis of patterns of communication. *American Journal of Public Health*, 1968, *58*, 274–288.

Evans, J. L. Psychiatric illness in the physician's wife. *American Journal of Psychiatry*, 1965, *122*, 159–163.

Fraser, F. C. Genetic counseling. *American Journal of Human Genetics*, 1974, *26*, 636–659.

Gillum, R. F. & Borsky, A. J. Diagnosis and management of patient noncompliance. *Journal of American Medical Association*, 1974, *228*, 1563–1567.

Goldstein, A. P. & Dean, S. J. *The investigation of psychotherapy*. New York: J. Wiley and Sons, 1966.

Kennedy, D. A. Perceptions of illness and healing. *Social Science and Medicine*, 1973, 7, 787–805.

Krell, R. & Miles, J. E. Marital therapy of couples in which the husband is a physician. *American Journal of Psychotherapy*, 1976, 30, 267–275.

Lappé, M. Allegiances of human geneticists: A preliminary typology. *Hastings Center Studies*, 1973, 1, 63–78.

London, P. *Behavior control*. New York: Harper and Row, 1969.

Maiman, L. A. & Becker, M. H. The health belief model: Origins and correlates in psychological theory. In M. H. Becker (Ed.), *The health belief model and personal health behavior*. Thorofare, New Jersey: Slack, 1974.

Parsons, T. *The social sytem*. New York: The Free Press, 1951.

Patterson, C. H. *Theories of counseling and psychotherapy*. New York: Harper and Row, 1966.

Siegler, M. & Osmond, H. *Models of madness, models of medicine*. New York: Macmillan, 1974.

Sorenson, J. R. Sociological and psychological factors in applied human genetics. In B. Hilton, D. Callahan, M. Harris, P. Condliffe & B. Berkley (Eds.), *Ethical issues in human genetics*. New York: Plenum Press, 1973.

Sorenson, J. R. Biomedical innovation, uncertainty, and doctor–patient interaction. *Journal of Health and Social Behavior*, 1974, 15, 366–374.

Szasz, T. S. & Hollender, M. H. A contribution to the philosophy of medicine: The basic models of the doctor–patient relationship. *Archives of Internal Medicine*, 1956, 97, 585–592.

Taviss, I. Problems in the social control of biomedical science and technology. In E. Mendelsohn, J. P. Swazey & I. Taviss, (Eds.), *Human aspects of biomedical innovation*. Cambridge: Harvard University Press, 1971.

Truax, C. B. & Carkhuff, R. R. *Introduction to counseling and psychotherapy: Training and practice*. Chicago: Aldine Press, 1966.

Vaillant, G. E., Sobowak, N. C. & McArthur, C. Some psychologic vulnerabilities of physicians. *New England Journal of Medicine*, 1972, 287, 372–375.

White, R. W. *The enterprise of living*. New York: Holt, Rinehart and Winston, 1972.

The Genetic Counseling Session 5

Seymour Kessler

In this chapter the genetic counseling process itself will be considered. Perforce, the views presented here will be highly personal ones. Each counselor has his or her own set of ideals, values, and needs which he or she will attempt to realize or fulfill in the genetic counseling session. Multiple paths might be taken to reach the same goal, and no argument will be made that the views advanced here should or ought to be adopted as *the* standard way of doing genetic counseling.

The kind of genetic counseling session described here is one in which the data gathering and diagnostic activities have been completed and, following some unspecified period of time and/or rituals to mark off the session from what preceded it, the counselors and counselees sit down together to discuss the diagnosis and its implications (including possible reproductive options) and attempt an integration. As practiced in different centers, genetic counseling may differ in some ways from this simplifying conceptual model. Hopefully, the reader will recognize sufficient points of contact between his or her own experiences and the present discussion and will be able to make the necessary extrapolations from one framework to another so that the discussion becomes personally meaningful.

Psychological issues are omnipresent in the genetic counseling session and the interventions made by the genetic counselor may be used to either facilitate or to inhibit their emergence. Usually, empathic statements and questions facilitate whereas nonempathic statements and questions inhibit the expression of these issues. It is largely a matter of

65

GENETIC COUNSELING
Psychological Dimensions

personal judgment when to be facilitative and when it is wiser not to be so. For example, in gathering specific medical data or family history, some counselors might deliberately choose to be nonfacilitative. If a counselee nevertheless shows strong feelings during this process, the counselor might then want to shift to a more facilitative mode of interaction rather than to defer dealing with these emotions to a later point in the session. One's intuitive sense is usually a reliable guide when to "pull" for psychological material; for the counselor who is not comfortable relying on intuition, trial-and-error learning may provide a handle on this issue.

Although there are commonalities in general outline from session to session, each genetic counseling session is a unique experience for the participants. Because of this it is impossible to advance a set of rules which are fully applicable to all circumstances. The genetic counselor, like any counselor or therapist, may need to face a range of ambiguities and unknowns in any given session and, in the final analysis, will need to make a series of on-the-spot assessments and judgments as to what course to steer. The ability to make such effective judgments is a function of experience and the extent of the counselor's flexibility in uncertain situations. Flexibility generally develops as a result of experiences in which the counselor has tried different approaches to somewhat similar tasks and has discovered what works "best" and under what conditions.

The Structure of the Genetic Counseling Session

The structure of the session is determined by multiple factors. Unlike the nondirective psychotherapeutic encounter, in which the conuselor-therapist assumes a relatively passive stance, the genetic counselor generally plays an active role in bringing structure to the session. Almost always, counselors come to the session with an agenda; they need to find out or recheck things about the counselees (e.g., details of family history) and, in turn, to transmit genetic, medical, and other information to them. To greater or lesser extent, these needs generally mesh with numerous other conscious and unconscious personal and professional needs and motives the counselors have. The counselees also come to the session with their agenda(s). They may want to obtain some specific information, and they may need help in understanding and making sense out of their experiences. Also, they often have needs to be reassured and validated by the counselor. Not infrequently, in their mind's eye, the counselees may have already lived through the session, as if to rehearse the experience. In such preparatory work, they may have worked out some formula of reassurance or restoration. For example, they may have imagined the counselor telling them, "Your unborn baby is definitely healthy," or they may fantasy the counselor undoing some past misfortune (e.g., "We have just discovered a miracle drug which cures Down syndrome," or, "We now have new evidence that the diagnosis given your child last year is incorrect; he is really normal."). Such fantasies, hopes, and wishes are like anchoring points (see page 44) from which the counselees evaluate whatever else occurs (or does not occur) in the session. Often, such fantasies are ungratified leading to a sense of disappointment that is reinforced by feeling foolish that one has allowed oneself to indulge in such fantasies.

As soon as the counselor and counselees meet, they begin to influence and shape each other's behavior and agendas in an attempt to have their respective needs met; in analyzing the content and process of the genetic counseling session, one is struck by the many subtle ways by which this occurs. Through the nuances of their interactions, each participant is striving to be heard, acknowledged, accepted, and validated.

The genetic counseling session may be divided into three major overlapping phases, a beginning or *initial contact* phase, a middle or *encounter* phase and an end or *summary* phase. Preceding the session itself, an *intake* phase generally occurs and, often, following the session, anywhere from minutes to months, a *followup* session or sessions may occur. Thus, in all, five phases will be discussed, each of which will be considered in turn. For the sake of simplifying the discussion, it will be assumed that the genetic counseling will be accomplished in a single session and that a male counselor, unless otherwise indicated, will be meeting with a husband and wife. In actual practice, departures from these conditions often occur. In some genetic counseling centers, diagnostic evaluations constitute a central part of the session in which counseling is provided, and/or multiple session counseling is practiced and, frequently, a team approach is used in which several different professionals are involved in the face-to-face counseling encounter. And, of course, not all genetic counselors are males and not all counselees are married. Optimally, genetic counseling occurs over a series of sessions. However, limited facilities and manpower as well as other priorities may diminish the ability of various centers to provide the services they might like to offer.

The Intake Phase

Intake procedures tend to set the tone of the subsequent counseling. In this phase, the initial contact between the genetic counseling clinic and the counselees or referring physician (or agency) is made. The contact may be made by letter, telegram, phone, or in person. In many centers, a secretary, nurse, genetic associate, or some other person other than the counselor is the first to discuss the counseling with the prospective counselees or their representatives.

The intake phase involves data gathering and assessment. Medical history and the facts regarding the genetic disorder, its distribution among family members, the confirmation of diagnoses, and so forth are generally obtained. Obtaining the family history and medical records provides the initial opportunities for the counselees to play an active role in their subsequent counseling. Each effort the counselees make, in calling or writing to other physicians and to institutions in order to obtain records for the genetic counseling clinic, is a step toward involvement. The clinic may want to provide the request or release forms, but allowing the counselees to fill out the forms and to address and mail the envelopes themselves encourages their activity, even though it appears, on the surface, to be a small point of consideration.

The intake phase may be a good point for the genetic counselors or their representative to talk over the phone to the couple (and possibly other family members) seeking counseling. It is probably less confusing for the prospective counselees if a minimum number of different persons from the clinic are involved in making contact with them. The more persons involved, the greater the risks for misunderstandings developing, which may interfere with the counselor's ability to provide adequate counseling later on. One of the more difficult situations that may occur in genetic counseling is the emergence of information or misinformation requiring the counselors to reconcile their own views with those of someone else not present during the counseling. The latter may be a colleague of the counselors' or the counselees' physician. Considerable tact is needed in such situations to avoid undermining the counselees' confidence in their physician or, for that matter, in the counselors and the clinic. Not infrequently, correct information may have been given earlier, but subsequently misunderstood or distorted by the counselees.

The intake phase also provides an opportunity to make a psychosocial assessment of the counselees. Careful attention needs to be given to what the counselees say and how they say it. Their responses to routine questions, the degree to which they take initiative on their own behalf, their eagerness (or lack thereof) to come for counseling are all statements of their needs and of who they are as individuals and as a couple. Above all, the counselors need to attend to how the counselees present themselves— as competent adults or as helpless children—as this provides clues as to the counseling tactics they may need to employ later on when the face-to-face meeting with them actually occurs.

Sometimes counselors return a telephone call requesting genetic counseling and find themselves being manipulated into providing the counseling over the phone. With experience, one can usually detect such persons early on in the conversation. The counselor might then make process statements, that is, reply to underlying metamessages rather than to requests for detailed information. In such circumstances the counselor needs to provide a message along the lines of: "I can hear your concern and I would like to help you reach some better understanding (of this disorder). However, I do not feel comfortable dealing with you in this impersonal way. I would be glad to meet with you and talk to you and help you in whatever way I can. I would like to suggest that you and your spouse talk it over, and if you decide that the two of you want to come to the clinic, I would be pleased to discuss this matter further."

The Initial Contact Phase

In this phase, the counselor and counselees actually meet in person. This phase is a relatively short one and frequently consists of apparently unrelated or insignificant chit-chat about the weather or other seemingly inconsequential matters. Such banter serves a "warmup" function for both counselor and counselees. Also, a number of things occur during this period which have important consequences for the counseling session. As in any other social situation in which strangers meet, the initial few minutes of contact are ones in which each person quickly "sizes up" the other, determines what the other person may expect of him or her, sends messages as to what is expected of the other person, and compares himself or herself to the other with respect to multiple dimensions (i.e., stronger–weaker, more or less intelligent, more or less attractive, etc.). In addition, the rules by which the transactions between the various parties will be carried out are established and the limits of the relationship are defined. Most of this is done in an implicit way. Also, it is in this phase that the counselors generally transmit to the counselees their expectations, "I expect you to be passive (or active)," thus establishing the general pattern of their relationship during the next hour or so.

In their mutual assessment, the counselor and counselee are attempting to determine the answer to one essential question, "Can I trust this person?" The primary task of the initial contact phase is the establishment of mutual trust. Failure to develop such feelings will interfere with the effectiveness of the counseling. The counselees will withhold their true feelings and, possibly, important pieces of (emotionally charged) information as well. Genetic and medical information provided by the counselor may be discounted or disbelieved. If the counselors perceive that they are being mistrusted, this may influence their feelings toward the counselees and interfere with their ability to provide information and to be empathic.

If the counselor's initial contact with the counselees occurs in the counseling session, clarification should be obtained from the counselees about their expectations of the meeting. By doing so, the counselor can ascertain the degree to which their agenda(s) interdigitate with his or her own.[1] A statement such as, "What is your understanding of why we are meeting today?" or some other equivalent open-ended inquiry may be a good way for the counselor to begin. A question of this sort may elicit a statement from the counselees consistent with the counselor's own expectations ("Oh, we are here to find out about our chances of having a child with cystic fibrosis."). The situation here is clear, as all participants have shared expectations. This may not always be the case. For example, in the following instance the counselor's opening question reveals incongruent expectations [2] :

C: What's your understanding of our getting together?
W: Hum. Um. I don't know.
C: (turns toward husband) And you, Mr. F., what's your understanding?
H: I'm not too sure.
C·   What was it Dr. A. told you when he referred you to the clinic here?

Generally a question of the latter sort begins to open things up. If it does not, the counselor will need to make a rapid assessment of the situation. Are the counselees overly suspicious or cautious persons? Are they playing "dumb" (a passive–aggressive ploy), or are they truly ignorant of the purpose of the meeting? If the counselor believes that they are indeed uninformed, he or she might then say to the counselees, "Well, my understanding of our meeting is . . . , etc." going on to explain what the counselor would like to accomplish and talk about. Before launching into the agenda, the counselor should first check out how the counselees

---

[1] A standard and useful counseling tactic is for the counselors to first elicit the attitudes, beliefs, expectations, and understandings of the counselees before advancing their agendas, answers, and explanations. This approach provides the counselors with a context for understanding the *meaning* of the counselees' questions. Even an apparently simple question may have multiple meanings and the counselors cannot assume, in the absence of clarifying data, that their understandings are those of the counselees. Also, some counselees are overly compliant and will not reveal their agendas and concerns once the counselor has stated his or her own. By facilitating the expression of the counselees' agenda, the counselor conveys messages of interest in their problems and confidence in their ability to manage their lives.

[2] C = counselor (male); C2 = counselor (female); H = husband; W = wife.

feel about the agenda and also how they managed to get this far and remain so uninformed. They may be truly naive and also angry at their physician (and possibly others) for not having been told why they were referred for genetic counseling.

The passive couple might be dealt with by saying something along the lines of, "Well, it certainly must be confusing to you to come all this way and not know why." This may lead to transactions which eventually may reveal the following:

CONTENT	PROCESS NOTES, COMMENTS AND HYPOTHESES
W: Well, we're here only because Dr. B. told us to come.	"We wouldn't be here on our own."
H: He wanted us to come here.	H sounds irritated.
C: It sounds to me that you are annoyed at him for suggesting that you come here.	C reflects back H's affective tone.
W: Yeah, I think he's making a mountain out of a molehill.	W is also annoyed at Dr. B.
H: Yeah.	
C: I'm wondering, now that you are here, whether or not you expect me to behave that way too.	Rather than explore their anger at Dr. B. further at this point, C retains the focus on the present task of establishing confidence and trust. Once trust is established, the "molehill" can be more effectively dealt with. The fact needs to be recognized that despite their feelings toward Dr. B., they did come to the counseling session so perhaps on some level, they too recognize their need to be there. C wants to avoid becoming either a defender of Dr. B. or of being placed into a position where C needs to judge who is right or wrong.

Interventions of this kind may expose the counselees' resistance or reluctance to engaging with the counselor in the work of the counseling. Generally, such couples are very anxious about what the counselor might say to them and thus use passivity as a defensive maneuver. If the counselor is empathic and provides them with a milieu of safety, they often let down their defensiveness and show a more pleasant, cooperative side.

Reluctance to engage fully in the counseling situation may be expressed by many different routes. Not infrequently the counselees may present themselves in such a way as if to deny the fact that *they* indeed are the counselees. For example, parents may explain that they have come for counseling on behalf of their children or some other relative rather than for themselves. They might say that *they* are not concerned; it is the child or the relative who is wondering about the recurrence risk or concerned about the disorder. Frequently, the thought that they are carriers of genes which have led (or may lead) to an affected child is anxiety provoking. Also, the information they anticipate that the counselor may convey is so threatening to such counselees that distancing from the problem is used as a defensive strategy.

Two common errors may be made in counseling such couples: (*a*) the counselor may call attention to the counselees' defensiveness too quickly thereby undermining it, or (*b*) it may be ignored altogether, generally because the counselor is unaware of the degree of their defensiveness. By undermining their defenses too quickly, the counselor may succeed in raising the counselees' defensiveness still further. This is generally non-productive as it may interfere with their ability to hear and understand the information the counselor needs to provide. At the initial point in their relationship with the counselor, the counselees are not ready to lower their guardedness. Thus, the counselor needs to allow their defensiveness at this point. However, once a counseling alliance has been solidified, the counselor will need to deal with the counselees' feelings and to assist them to acknowledge the fears and apprehensions they have previously externalized. Without this step, the counselees may not be able to integrate most effectively the material received from the counselor.

A brief example follows. An autosomal recessive disorder is involved and only the mother of the affected child (Sally) is present with the counselor in the session. Sally's older sister is now 12 years of age. The following exchange occurs early in the session:

C: I wonder if you have specific questions you want me to address myself to?

W: Well, my daughter will need to begin to think about having children of her own and what should be done. She'll be dating soon and what approach should she take. How soon should she tell someone about it and what are her chances of having a normal baby? — *W is acting as an agent for her daughter. This should alert C to a possibly high level of defensiveness.*

C: Has she been asking you questions about Sally's problems?

W: No, she never does. It's just that I suddenly realized that she is growing up. — *One wonders what has happened to make her aware that her child is no longer a child. Perhaps the daughter has begun to menstruate.*

C: It sounds like your daughter is no — *C attempts to form an identification be-*

longer a little child for you. Before you know it, she'll be having children of her own.

tween mother and daughter, so that as he deals with the issue of the latter passing "bad" genes on to her progeny, he simultaneously helps W to work through her own feelings on this issue.

Later, as the session progressed and the relationship between C and W solidified, W was able to admit that there was much that *she* did not understand about the disorder. It then became possible to deal with the issue of what it meant for her to be the carrier of genes which led to an affected child. During the course of this discussion C pointed out that perhaps the thought that she had passed a gene on to her daughter which might result in further affected children was too distressing for her to deal with when the session began.

With suspicious couples, until their suspicions are verbalized and scrutinized by the counselor and counselees, it would be a mistake to continue on to the next phase of the counseling. Often, virtually everyone with whom such counselees have had contact in arranging the counseling may have become drawn into the web of their suspicions. Confusion generally results. Chance remarks and seemingly insignificant events may be converted into vague, yet meaningful, bits of data providing support for their highly personal beliefs. The possibility that the counselor knows something about them that they do not is particularly threatening to them. Thus, they may be hostile to the counselor, evasive and strongly defended against what the counselor may have to say.

In the transcript that follows, a suspicious couple will be considered. The couple has been referred for preamniocentesis counseling because of maternal age. Both H and W are well educated and have been married about 6 years. A routine family history has been obtained by phone by Dr. D., of the clinic staff, several days prior to the counseling.

C: What's your undertanding about our meeting today?

Addressed to both H and W.

H: I would like maybe for you to explain more about it. I'm not sure exactly what you do and . . . (breaks off).

H is guarded. His use of the word "maybe" suggests that he may be ambivalent about being here. The fact that he abruptly fails to complete his last sentence suggests that he will not put out more than he has to. One might speculate that he was going to say, "I'm not sure what you do and what you want from me."

C: So you don't have a clear picture to focus on?

H: No.

Again, H is not too communicative.

C: (Turns to W) And how about you?

C's statement is deliberately unstructured

W: Um. No. I really don't have a clear picture of what you plan to say. One of the things I would like to know is what made Dr. D. decide that we should come in?

and is being used as a probe to uncover the source of H's cautiousness.

Like H, W is being very cautious. Note her use of C's phrase, ". . . don't have a clear picture. . . ." The participants have only been together a few moments and a subtle influence of one person's behavior on the other's has already occurred.

C: Dr. D?

C is caught by surprise and is puzzled.

W: Yes, Dr. D.

C: You were referred to the clinic, so fas as I can see, by Dr. E . . .

Confusion is becoming apparent.

W: (Interrupts) But . . .

C: . . . and, um, yeah, go ahead.

W: Okay, when I talked to Dr. E's nurse and then when I initially talked to Dr. D., I had the feeling that he didn't think that there would be too much point in our coming in here. But then at some point when I was giving him all the information, he apparently changed his mind. What is it that may have changed it?

W does not say that Dr. D. told her that there was no point in coming in, she only says that it was her *feeling* that that was what he had intended to say. Perhaps Dr. D. was not as clear as he could have been. Nevertheless, W appears to want to believe that there is something about herself that required the adoption of procedures outside the usual routine.

C: (Cautiously) I'm not quite sure . . .

C has become as guarded as the counselees were earlier.

C has several options open to him at this point. He might ask W to reconstruct her conversation with Dr. D. and then try to undermine her belief that Dr. D. had changed his mind. This tactic may be difficult to accomplish and may place C in the position of being a judge. Another approach would be to say, "I really don't know what Dr. D. or Dr. E's nurse said to you and most certainly what they had in mind. All I can do is to start from scratch, review your family and medical history, etc.," and then go on to propose a contract for the forthcoming session. Lastly, and perhaps the best strategy, C might reflect back the counselees' apparent lack of enthusiasm about being there for counseling and then explore what it means for them to actually be there.

In this case, C adopted none of these strategies. Rather, he attempted to reassure the counselees that their referral to the clinic was a routine one based on the fact that W is now 35 years of age. C then went on to lay out his agenda and proceeded to recheck family history and launched into content material. Forty or so minutes later, the following exchange occurred:

C: Do you have any other questions I can answer for you at this point?

W: What in our background made it seem as if it would be a better idea to come in for counseling? There's nothing you can say on that?

W has not been reassured by C's explanations. She continues to believe that something is being withheld from her. It is as if everything between the beginning of the session and now has not occurred for her.

By this time, both counselor and counselees are somewhat frustrated. C suggests that perhaps Dr. D should be invited to join the session and one might have thought that W would have welcomed this opportunity to clear up any of her lingering doubts and misconceptions. Surprisingly, W strongly resisted this idea. From her viewpoint, bringing in Dr. D. exposed her to the risk of being shown to be wrong and thus humiliated especially after already having made such a "fuss." It appeared to be important to her to hold on to the belief that she was being victimized. Perhaps this legitimized her anger at the clinic staff for exposing her to thoughts that frightened or distressed her (e.g., the amniocentesis procedure, abortion, the possibility of a defective fetus, etc.).

Sometimes, couples are hostile or suspicious because they perceive antagonism or dislike directed at them by the counselor. One question genetic counselors might ask themselves in the initial phase of the session is, "Do I like these people (the counselees)?" Obviously, it is impossible to like everyone and just as obviously we react differently to persons we like than to those we do not. To be effective, the counselors need to understand what it is about themselves that makes them tend to react to certain people in one way and to others dissimilarly.

The Middle or Encounter Phase

The heart of the genetic counseling session is the middle or encounter phase. It is here that the counselor imparts information, discusses genetic and medical matters, deals with the emotional reactions of the counselees and assists them to reach decisions on health and reproductive issues. The discussion below will be organized around several issues: rechecking the family history, determining the level of knowledge of factual material, providing information, dealing with marital dysfunctions, dealing with guilt feelings, and helping the counselees to make decisions. Major attention will be given to the issues of marital problems, guilt feelings and decision making.

The encounter phase may be an appropriate time to recheck the details of the counselees' family history. Unwanted pregnancies, miscarriages, and deaths of close relatives may be brought up along with painful memories and unresolved conflicts. Strong emotions may be expressed, although this is less likely to occur if the counselor is a stranger to the counselees. More likely, the counselees' eyes may well up, their voices may crack, and other signs of distress and emotional turmoil may be displayed. The trustworthiness of the counselor will be tested here ("Is this person someone with whom it is safe to share our feelings?"). The counselor would do well to respond empathically to the counselees at this point. Statements like, "This seems to be painful for you," "You must have loved your father very much," and other sincere, appropriate signs of empathy help to strengthen the relationship with the counselees and convey the message that the counselor cares about them and their feelings and that the counselor is willing to listen to their inner pain.

If the counselees have myths regarding their own health or that of other family members, these may emerge when the counselor rechecks the family history. Elaborate and sometimes improbable details regarding purported diagnoses and symptoms may be presented to the counselor with total certitude. This may not be the time to contradict, deflate, or correct these misconceptions; the counselor may not yet have important pieces of information bearing on the role such myths may play in the counselees' overall system of beliefs. Instead, the counselor should mentally file the major details of the myths and, if appropriate, deal with them later in the session when, presumably, the counselor–counselee relationship has been strengthened.

As the middle phase progresses, the counselor will begin to deal with the specific genetic disorder and its mode of inheritance. Before doing so, it is often worthwhile to explore the counselees' degree of understanding of genetics and of other pertinent factual information. In doing so, the counselor has another opportunity to promote the active participation of the counselees in the session. It is important that their participation be a rewarding experience. Some counselors favor the use of catethetic or classroom tactics. These give the appearance of evoking counselee involvement. In reality, such approaches tend to infantilize them and foster their passivity; some of the pitfalls of these approaches are evident in the following transcript:

C:	O.K. Do you know what chromosomes are?	A question in this format tends to pull for a "Yes" or "No" answer and thus is relatively nonfacilitating of further communication. An example of a more facilitative question is: "What's your understanding of chromosomes?"
H:	Uh huh.	A noncommital "Yes."
C:	Can you tell me what they are?	
H:	Well, they are part of the genes	

that determine what a person will look like and what their intelligence will be and things like that. They get half of them from the mother and half from the father.

C: For that, you get a good grade. You got the half-and-half.
(Everyone laughs)
(Turns to W): How would you define them?

C's rewarding statement is said good-naturedly; nevertheless, its content underscores the childlike position into which the counselees have been placed.

W: I would say that they are a basic unit of cells and they foretell how each cell is developing.

C: That's pretty good. You're both right. (C goes on to talk about genes and chromosomes.)

C rewards W, but compared to the one accorded H only a moment ago, it is of relatively lesser impact. C concludes the reward to W by rewarding H again. Such differential validation is likely to lead to W becoming more and more passive.

C may be more comfortable with H than with W. He may see her as assertive or threatening and may have negative feelings toward her. Unconsciously, he might feel more comfortable if she were less active in the session.

The transcript which follows concerns the same couple, but at an earlier point in the session. C is again trying to determine the counselees' baseline level of knowledge, this time about Down Syndrome. In the process of doing so, C establishes the pattern of interactions, evident in the previous transcript, in which he plays the parental role and the counselees play the role of children. The system of differential payoffs to H and W is also seen, but, here we will see how the counselees are complicit in sustaining this system. It is as if one of the family rules by which the counselees live is that the needs of the husband have priority over those of the wife.

C: Do you know what Down's Syndrome is?

The question is directed to both counselees.

W: I just think of those children I know who have it.

W responds first. She is responding "Yes" to C's question, "I know children with DS and I have thoughts about them." C might ask at this point, "And what comes to mind about DS children?" or, "What thoughts do you have about those children?" Such questions are facilitating ones as they open the way for the counselees to share their knowledge and thoughts.

C: What come to mind? What single condition within all the constellation of things that they have? What's the one condition that really strikes you the most?

Multiple questions tend to lead to confusion. C's opening question is a facilitating one. However, the question that follows tends to channel the counselee's awareness away from her own thoughts to those of C. W is in the position of needing to guess what C has in mind. The third question in this group again asks W to share what really strikes her the most about DS children. W now needs to reconcile conflicting demands: "Does he want me to tell him what *I* really think or does he want me to guess what *he* thinks about DS?"

W: That they are very puffy, have a large forehead and their eyes protrude.

W tells C what strikes *her* the most about DS children.

C: What is it that bothers you the most about Down's Syndrome?

C does not validate W's answer, rather he continues to probe for a different answer. C is assuming that what bothers him the most will also be the thing that bothers W the most about DS.

W: Um, the children aren't normal, and they wouldn't live a normal life.

W's reaction time is slowing down. She knows that she is familiar with DS yet she seems to be unable to guess what C has on his mind. She is becoming more cautious as the confidence in her knowledge is undermined.

C: Why wouldn't they? What is it about? What is it?

C is becoming more insistent; his questions are shorter in length and structurally incomplete, for example, he is really asking, "What is it about DS that does not permit DS children to live a normal life?"

W: Um
C: What is the defect?

W is stalling; she may be confused.
C is now aware of W's "confusion" and is beginning to cue her by introducing the word, "defect."

H: (turns to W) we were talking about that last night.

Rather than answer C's question, H joins into the "Guess What I'm Thinking" game on C's side to provide a cue to W. It is now two against one in the game, two men against a woman.

W: When?

W does not seem to know what is expected of her.

H: Their mind.

After permitting W to flounder awhile, H now comes to her rescue. His response is peculiarly vague.

C: That's right. That's what I'm really fishing for. That's fine, their mind. They are mentally retarded.

C admits that he had something specific in mind all along. "That's right" and "That's fine," are rewarding statements, that is, rewards for a correct answer. As played here, the game of "Guess What I'm Thinking" has a benign tone. Nevertheless, it does have an impact on the players. Most often the person in the child's role ends up feeling stupid or incompetent. As played here, this game tends to emphasize the power differential between the counselor and the counselees; C is the knowing parent, and H and W are the children. It is important to note that although W has been supplying good answers to C's questions, it is H who receives the reward in the end. In its more pernicious form, this game is one of the ways sexism is experienced by some women.

W: Oh, I see. That's right.

It is not clear what W sees. She may be saying, "I see now what you were fishing for." She sounds embarrassed.

C: Yes, that's the point I wanted to make with you to get a start. [C goes on to explain the retardation and other phenotypic manifestations of DS.] Have you seen children with DS?

W: I've seen like two, where I work.

C: [Describes the facial features and similarity of appearance of DS children.]

C does not acknowledge W's statement or her experience. He addresses himself to the description of DS children as if he had heard W say, "I've seen two and they looked alike." Such mental transformations are not uncommon in the counseling session. Sometimes, as here, they have a poetic quality.

H: I've only seen pictures of them.

H has less direct experience with DS than W.

C: [Continues to describe the features of DS children.] DS is a host of birth defects, not just mental retardation. But the biggest impact is mental retardation.

H: That's the one that bothers me the most.

H may be attempting to cement an alliance with C by responding to C's previous question ("What bothers you the most about DS?") at this point. Despite the fact that several transactions have occurred, H has held back from making a forthright statement of what bothers him until now, only after C has explained his own position. One might

> hypothesize that H is particularly cautious
> in unknown situations, that he has strong
> needs for being seen by others as intelli-
> gent and as not making mistakes. Thus,
> he may hold back until he is sure of how
> others feel before committing himself
> to a point of view. He may, therefore,
> have difficulty making autonomous
> decisions.

As a general rule, as soon as possible after new information is conveyed to the counselees, especially that regarding diagnostic and genetic risk issues, the counselor should inquire what this information means to the counselees. Questions such as, "I wonder what thoughts you have about what I just told you?" or "How do you feel about what I've said?" provide a glimpse of how the information is being processed cognitively and affectively so that its later integration can be facilitated. By inquiring, the counselor conveys the message that he respects the counselees by being aware that the information is affecting them. Replies such as, "I don't know," should be pursued with questions such as, "I wonder what your first impressions are?". I have gone as far as saying, "I'm puzzled about the fact that you have no feelings about (reaction to) the informa- tion I gave you. I know that if it was me on the receiving end, I would be upset (overjoyed) to hear . . . etc." Some counselors are reluctant to interfere with the flow of their agenda by making such inquiries and allowing the counselees space to react to highly charged information until some predetermined point later in the session. This is certainly preferable to not eliciting their reactions at all. However, it is less preferable than a style of counseling which recognizes and acknowledges feelings as they occur and which allows counselor and counselees to interact more freely and spontaneously.

Providing a genetic risk figure should be made as simply as possible. Few counselees are interested in the degree of mathematical precision that most geneticists attempt to achieve when they calculate genetic risks. Those who do engage the counselor in a detailed discussion of risk gen- erally do so as a means of avoiding (or controlling) the emotions evoked by such discussions. A formulation such as follows, although accurate, is stylistically too complex and ought to be avoided:

C: I believe the chances of this happen-
    ing again are no greater than one in
    a hundred. The other way of looking
    at it means, of course, that better
    than 99 chances out of a 100, the
    baby won't have this condition.

A simple statement, like, "I believe that the chances of this happening again are one in a 100, that is, 1%; that means that 99% of the time it won't happen again," will suffice. This might be followed immediately by a question along the following lines: "I wonder how you hear that?"

One of the more difficult moments in genetic counseling involves the provision of a recurrence risk for conditions in which the heritable nature and risk of recurrence are obscure (e.g., conditions in which one cannot distinguish the possibility of a phenocopy from a dominant mode of inheritance and for which information on the proportion of all cases which are genetically determined is lacking). In effect, the counselors need to say in all honesty that they do not know what the recurrence risk is for a particular couple. The counselees are often disappointed that unequivocal information cannot be supplied and not infrequently will become angry at the counselor. Under such circumstances, it is necessary to be empathic and supportive of their feelings (e.g., "I guess if I were in your place, I'd be angry too.").

In general, giving the same risk figure from two perspectives (25% chance of an affected and 75% chance of a normal baby) is a good idea as it is less "leading." However, careful judgment needs to be exercised in specific cases. Some counselors prefer to support a decision they perceive the counselees have already made by phrasing the risk figure in such a way as to emphasize or de-emphasize the chances of having an affected child.

After providing a genetic risk figure, the counselor might inquire, "I wonder what a one in four (or other appropriate figure) risk means for you?" or, "Some couples feel that a one chance out of four is a low risk whereas others feel it is a high risk. I wonder how you feel about it?" Responses to such inquiries frequently reveal the meanings counselees give to the information provided by the counselor.

MARITAL DYSFUNCTIONS

Dysfunctional relationships often become evident during the genetic counseling session. The extent to which genetic counselors would want to deal with these interpersonal problems is largely a function of personal preference and predilection, time priorities and their competence in doing so. Often the relationship problems have a clear impact on their ability to provide genetic information or to help the counselees reach pertinent reproductive or health decisions. In such cases, the counselors may be remiss by not intervening in a therapeutic way, even if this only means that they point out or identify the problem for the counselees and refer them to an appropriate professional. Needless to say, appropriate training

in crisis intervention and/or family therapy is a prerequisite to effective
and lasting interventions.

Two of the major signs of a dysfunctional relationship are poor interpersonal communication and the absence of adequate means of conflict
resolution. Dysfunctional communication is often manifested by an interpersonal style in which the counselees conspicuously do not make contact.
Literally, eye contact may be noticeably absent. Often the couple tends
to talk past each other. Statements are made in the form of questions,
and questions go unanswered. Verbalizations are unclear, indirect, and
vague, and the various levels of communication are incongruent. There
is a lack of respect for and little acknowledgement of the worth of the
other. One's ability to talk, to finish a sentence, to emote and to respond
to third parties may all be interfered with. In the counseling session,
divergent views on important issues may emerge to the mate's surprise;
a basic lack of trust may interfere with their ability to discuss such issues
beforehand.

Two persons involved in a long-term relationship must in time come
to deal with areas of disagreement and conflict. In the absence of mechanisms to resolve conflicts, a dysfunctional relationship invariably results.
For example, the emergence of longstanding grudges during the course
of genetic counseling suggests that the couple has difficulties resolving
conflict. In counseling such couples, the counselors need to be aware that
their attempts to reach closure on reproductive or health decisions may
be frustrated. Also, as they attempt to reach such closure, the counselors
may be unwittingly exacerbating an already existing schism between the
couple by their possibly taking one partner's side against the other.

The presence of unshared secrets and attempts to enlist the counselor's
assistance in maintaining a family secret may be another indicator of
marital dysfunction. If the counselors elect to participate with one counselee in maintaining a secret from the other, they need to realize that
their ability to help the counselees may be significantly curtailed. They
also risk losing the capacity to develop trust in their relationship with
them.

Relationships in which secrets play a part are often dominated by
feelings of shame and/or impotence and powerlessness; the secret provides a sense of defensive power and control. However, considerable and
continual effort needs to be expended to avert the exposure of the secret.
Thus, the system of rules and beliefs upon which such relationships are
based becomes less and less flexible and more incapable of changing over
time. A sense of power is bought through the loss of actual power. By
buying their belief system, the counselor may become as powerless as the
counselees.

Secrets and other indicators of marital dysfunction often emerge in the counseling session because the family system and the individuals in that system are generally under stress. When secrets do come out, they are almost invariably accompanied by intense feelings of anger and shame. The counselor and/or other clinic personnel may be targets of displaced rage. The fee charged for the counseling is a frequent target for such feelings. In general, high levels of anxiety or hostility and other seemingly "inappropriate" expressions of affect are often displacements of feelings that the counselees may have toward each other. The counselor may need to help them express these intense feelings toward the more appropriate object and to place matters in their proper perspective.

GUILT FEELINGS

The genetic counselor may play an active role in helping the counselees come to grips with their feelings of guilt. Despite the belief fostered in the genetic counseling literature that the counselor, through reassurances and corrections of misinformation, has the capacity to alleviate, diminish, lift, or otherwise alter guilt feelings, the reality is that the counselor has little power to absolve others of such feelings. This point might be better understood if we examine briefly the nature of guilt.

Two types of guilt might be differentiated, one based on a fear of punishment and the other, true guilt, which, according to Angyl (1965) involves a betrayal of somebody or something one loves. Related to the former are guilt feelings originating in an assumption of responsibility for events over which the person has no realistic control. It might be thought that such feelings might be alleviated when the counselor corrects the misconceptions upon which the guilt feelings are based. Unfortunately, such feelings are often intertwined with true guilt, and attempts to assuage, minimize, or cite extenuating circumstances are generally not effective in easing the counselees' feelings. Telling counselees that they did nothing for which they should feel guilty is not an effective way of dealing with their feelings. On the contrary, such statements convey the message that their feelings are not legitimate, or, worse, possibly abnormal. This should not be taken to mean that the counselor should not attempt to correct misinformation or misconceptions. Of course, the counselor should. However, such corrections need to be coupled with an acceptance of the counselees' feelings; reassuring them or otherwise using the counselor's status or prestige as a means of altering their feelings seldom has the effect the counselor intends. Reassurances are most often nonempathic and worse, statements of rejection.

In the same vein, discussing the ubiquitousness of the mutation process or the concept of lethal-equivalents provides little solace for the person who feels responsible for having conceived or given birth to a "defective" child. Such discussions generally inform the counselees that the intensity of their feelings has escaped the counselor.

Guilt brings both counselor and counselees face-to-face with an existential dilemma. To feel guilty implies that one had the capacity to alter events. The thought that if one had acted differently, one might have averted the birth of an affected child suggests that there were choices to be made and that one had the power to make a different choice. To argue that the person is not guilty for the birth of a "defective" child carries the implication that one was indeed powerless to alter events. To many, the prospect of having to face one's existential powerlessness and helplessness is far more distressing or frightening than a sense of guilt, which, after all, affirms the belief that one is potent. Most often, this all occurs on an unconscious level.

There are several general approaches the genetic counselor might use to deal with guilt feelings. From least to most effective, that is, from passive to active counselee participation, they are as follows:

1. The counselor might say to the counselees that they need not, ought not, or should not feel guilty. In this approach the counselor attempts to use the authority as a professional to influence the counselees' attitudes and beliefs. The counselor shares nothing of his or her own inner psychological world and is minimally involved interpersonally with the counselees. Presumably, because no demands are made of the counselees to invest their energy in confronting and working on their feelings, little long-term change in attitudes, beliefs, and feelings can be expected. One major pitfall of this approach is that it may actually increase a sense of guilt because it may make the person feel that the feelings are grossly inappropriate and thus one needs to feel guilty about feeling guilty.

2. The counselor might undermine distorted or mistaken beliefs and defensive denial and then verbalize, sympathetically, what he or she believes the counselees are feeling and thinking. In this approach, the counselor attempts to use rational arguments to influence the counselees' attitudes, beliefs, and feelings. Some demands are put on the counselees to deal with their feelings, but, on the whole, it is the counselor who does the major portion of the psychological work. A possible pitfall of this approach is that it may require the counselees to acknowledge feelings or give up defenses before they are ready to do so. This may lead to the appearance of "relief" in the immediate situation but also to a tightening up of the defenses that may interfere with their ability to work through their feelings in the long run.

3. The counselor might help the counselees to verbalize their own

feelings and thoughts and then to empathize with their feelings of guilt, remorse, and/or shame or with their sense of helplessness to alter or to have altered events. In this approach the responsibility for the psychological work rests with the counselees. The counselor acts as a facilitator and helps them to get in touch with, identify, and label their feelings. Because it is *their* energy invested in dealing with their feelings, whatever changes that occur are experienced as being a product of their own efforts and thus likely to be better integrated and maintained over time. At no time do the counselors imply that the counselees should feel differently than they do. On the contrary, they provide legitimization for the counselees' feelings. The counselors accept their feelings and convey the message that, even if in their own eyes they are imperfect, deficient and guilty, in theirs, they remain acceptable and worthy persons. In this approach the counselors must be completely involved with the counselees; they must be genuine, patient, accepting, empathic, and willing to be aware of and, if necessary, ready to share of their own inner experience.

In some situations in genetic counseling, the attempt to alleviate guilt would, in my opinion, be most inappropriate. For example, the attempt to diminish the guilt feelings of a mother of a child with fetal alcohol syndrome would not be supported by the reality of the situation. If the drinking behavior was maintained, it probably would be more therapeutic to promote the use of the guilt as a motivator for more adaptive behavior.

Before leaving the topic of guilt, one special group of couples, for whom issues of guilt may be especially prominent, should be mentioned; these are first cousins. Although some social groups condone or tolerate marriages between such relatives, other groups do not. It is important to explore with such couples how their respective families reacted to their plans to wed and/or to have children. Not infrequently, such couples have married despite family opposition. Thus, having a child, a healthy child, has special psychological meanings for such couples. When the issues are explored, some couples express strong feelings of guilt that they have acted contrary to parental and moral strictures and have unusual expectations that a deformed child will be their ultimate punishment. The possibility that first cousins may actually have a higher than average risk for a child with a congenital malformation exacerbates the fears that such will be their fate.

DECISION MAKING

Helping the counselees reach appropriate decisions is a process which begins from their initial contact with the genetic counseling clinic. The counselor has several tasks to accomplish to facilitate this process:

1. The counselor needs to help the counselees play an active role in their counseling. In many instances, the counselees have either placed themselves or have been placed into a relatively passive role with respect to their past relationships with medical professionals. The counselor needs to help the counselees to move from this state of mind to a more active psychological place. The paradox of the counseling encounter, as opposed to other professional or social relationships, is that when the counselor is overly authoritative, informative, and knowledgeable, he or she sets up unattainable standards for the counselees and thus impedes the development of the self-confidence needed to make rational, autonomous decisions. It is as if the counselor is conveying the message, "I am so wise that I can see better than you can what is best for you." The point at which the counselor becomes "too much" will vary from case to case; optimal levels need to be determined by the counselor's empathic sense.

Actions, interventions, and tactics of the genetic counselor or counseling team which involve the counselees in the session, facilitate the sharing of their thoughts and feelings and which address and evoke their adult side (Berne, 1964), will generally foster a psychologically active place. The psychologically active person has what Rotter (1966) terms an internal locus of control, that is, the person expects, perceives, and interprets personally meaningful events as being contingent upon his or her own behavior or personality rather than being the result of chance, luck, or fate or under the control of powerful others.

2. The counselor needs to raise pertinent issues, so that the counselees are informed, if they do not already know, what important problems they might anticipate by making (or not making) specific decisions. For example, in some genetic disorders there is a variable phenotypic expression of the mutant gene(s). If the counselees' experience is that the disorder manifests itself only in a mild way, they may not have a realistic appreciation of how severely affected an affected child might be, should they decide to reproduce. If (or once) they are informed, the counselor may participate with them in discussing what the decision may mean for them.

3. The counselor needs to point out options about which the counselees are unfamiliar or uninformed. This might include informing them of the availability of diagnostic procedures, artificial insemination, community resources, and so on, which might help them see their situation in a broader perspective.

4. Counselors need to help the counselees obtain a better understanding of the factors that impede their decision-making process. Often, important life decisions evoke ambivalent feelings. The counselors might point this out when such feelings become evident in the counseling session. Then they might help them explore the personal meaning each

side of the ambivalence has for them, as well as the function that the ambivalence plays in impeding their reaching closure on whatever needs to be decided.

Under most circumstances, counselees should make their own decisions regarding abortion, reproduction, and so forth. Some counselees may appear to be pleased to have a decision taken out of their hands. In the long run, however, decisions made by the counselor for the counselees reinforce their sense of inadequacy, incompetence, and helplessness. In helping the counselees reach a decision, the counselor needs to play the role of a guide and facilitator. The counselor needs to assess the direction of their thinking, point out pitfalls, and prepare the counselees for possible future problems. Questions such as, "I'm wondering whether or not you have given any thought to what you might do if the test showed that the baby was affected?" or, "Have you thought about what it might mean for you to go through a therapeutic abortion?", or some of those suggested in the transcripts below tend to facilitate the mutual exploration of issues.

Some of the factors contributing to requests or demands being made of the counselor to make a decision or to provide advice about various courses of action are as follows:

1. Good rapport between the counselor and counselees has not been established and mutual expectations have not been explored (e.g., a perceived need to be passive has been reinforced by the counselor).
2. The counselees experience the counselor as pressing for a decision before they are ready to reach closure.
3. The counselees are confused and/or do not understand the session content (e.g., information overload).
4. The presence of marital dysfunctions (e.g., counselees cannot agree and want a third party to take responsibility for a decision and/or to obtain an ally for their point of view).
5. Personality variables. For different reasons, both obsessives and hysterics might have difficulty reaching decisions and may wish or expect the counselor to make decisions for them.[3]

[3] Persons with an obsessive personality style tend to be perfectionistic and orderly (Shapiro, 1965). Their behavior is motivated largely by the need to obtain or sustain control over themselves and their environment in order to avoid feelings of helplessness and insecurity. Making mistakes or showing emotion are experienced as a loss of control by such individuals. They tend to use isolation of affect and intellectualization as major defenses. Reaching decisions is a difficult task for the obsessive because decisions often require taking a stand or making a commitment either to a person or a specific course of action (Salzman, 1973). This exposes the obsessive to the possibility of being wrong or making an error of judgment. Thus, they will tend to vacillate, procrastinate, and

6. The counselees are mentally retarded or otherwise incompetent to make decisions on their own.

The presence of one or more of the factors enumerated above may be sufficient to lead to such questions as, "What would you do in our place, doctor?" or (the more subtle), "Do most couples in our situation have this procedure?" Sometimes the latter question precedes the former one, in which case the counselor might reply, "Some couples decide to have it and others do not. You and your spouse will need to consider carefully all the facts and decide for yourselves what course of action is the best one for the two of you to take." Thus the counselor informs them that it is a couple's decision to make, not either one alone, and certainly not the counselor's. The counselor might go on to inquire, "I'm wondering what thoughts the two of you have given to this decision?" If they have not had an opportunity to talk it over yet, the counselor might suggest, "Well, here's your chance," or alternatively, suggest that they need to do so before they reach a decision and that he or she would be willing to help them in the areas in which they get stuck.

Like all other situations in counseling, there are appropriate moments for counselors to express their personal opinions, always keeping in mind that what they state will almost invariably be heard as a prescription for specific actions, not as personal opinion.

Some counselors respond to the question, "What do most couples do in our situation?" by providing information as to the modal behavior of other couples in similar circumstances. Such responses inform the counselee as to what appears to be appropriate and normal but does not address

---

to doubt, rationalizing their behavior as judicious scrutiny of all probabilities. Often, they make decisions by default; by delaying decision, circumstances or others take the decision into their own hands. If the decision turns out badly, they can shrug off responsibility and blame others or fate. When joint decisions are required, as they often are in genetic counseling, obsessives often evade being active participants in the decision-making process. Instead, they may appear to lend gracious support to whatever decision their partner might want to make. If things go wrong, they will not be in a position where they will be blamed.

Persons with a hysteric personality style tend to view the world in an impressionistic or diffuse way (Shapiro, 1965; MacKinnon & Michels, 1971). In contrast to the obsessive, hysterics tend to rely on affective truth (e.g., hunches, feelings), rather than on facts and logic as a way of relating to the world. They are easily distractible and impressionable. They generally use repression and denial as major defense mechanisms. Their feelings tend to be labile, sometimes volatile, but most often shallow and histrionic. In relating to men, female hysterics tend to act childlike and unconsciously manipulative and seductive. Whereas the obsessive tends to react unemotionally in situations of stress, hysterics respond as if they were helpless and overwhelmed. In this psychological place, the hysteric would have obvious difficulties making important life decisions.

what may be appropriate for *their* specific needs. Providing such information may, for some couples, actually make it more difficult for them to make a decision in their own self-interest.

Some of the major issues discussed above will be illustrated in the transcripts that follow. In the first one, a couple, in their mid-20s is being counseled following the birth of a pair of twins with multiple congenital defects. Only one of the babies, Ann, survived the perinatal period. As the transcript begins, we are somewhere in the middle of the encounter phase.

C: Let me ask you a question. At this point, do you know how many children you want?

C is attempting to explore the area of reproductive decisions. His question is too specific and will lead to eliciting facts rather than attitudes. A better inquiry might have been, "What thoughts have you given to having more children?"

W: Well, I'd like one more. I'd like . . .
C: (Interrupts) So you'd like to try again, huh?
W: Yeah.
C: How about you, Mr. Green?
H: How about, I'm not really eager to have any more . . . (mumbles).

H begins to repeat C's question. This may be a stalling tactic. H and W disagree about the question of more children.

C: Why is that?
H: Well, mostly financially. We want to buy a house. I don't want to have any more kids, that was, you know 'til we get into a house and see if we can afford it. That's the main reason for me (voice trails off).

H attempts to minimize the impact of the defective child; he says that it is *mostly* a question of money. He begins to say that he doesn't want to have another child with defects, but pulls back from actually stating it. He tends to use denial as a major means of defense.

C: How about Ann's condition? Does that have anything to do with your not being so eager to have more kids?

C picks up on the fact that H has backed off from mentioning Ann's defects as a reason for postponing further procreation. Note he asks about her "condition" not her "defects."

H: Uh, that's part of it too (half laughs).

H again minimizes the child's impact on his thinking and actions. C's question makes him anxious. One might speculate that, had C used the word, "defects," H would have denied C's question altogether. Wisely, C used the less-threatening word.

W: When she gets sick like this, you know, and stuff, she . . .

W hears H's anxiety and comes in to rescue him. One might conjecture that this couple will tend to unite in the face of an external threat. W may have difficulty dealing with H's anxiety and may work together with him to support a possible myth that he is the "strong" one in this family. W's statement also raises a question as to whether she really does want another child herself. It is unfortunate that C had interrupted her earlier statement on this matter.

H: (Simultaneously) She might still need more surgery.

W: Yeah.

W breaks off her own thought to agree with H.

C: Really, for the rectum and anus?

H and W: Yeah.

A moment ago it seemed as if H and W disagreed with each other over having more children. Now they seem to be in concert against C's efforts to uncover the feelings underlying their apparent disagreement. One wonders what C must be feeling now.

H: So far it looks good that she won't need it.

C: Dr. G told you that?

H: Yeah.

C: Have you run up a lot of bills that you have to pay for out of your own pocket?

H: Well, not very much. [He was in the military service when the child was born.]

C attempts to respond empathically to H's earlier statement regarding the financial impact of their child's defects. This statement raises some questions about H's earlier argument that financial considerations are the major reason for postponing reproduction.

C: Now, Mrs. Green, let me ask you this: What, at this time, what are the things that go through your mind when you look at Ann? What goes through your mind in terms of what's wrong with her? What conditions does she have?

C shifts gears abruptly. This may be a response to possible feelings of being shut out earlier by the counselees' coalition. He is attempting to determine how the counselees have integrated their knowledge of Ann's condition. A series of questions are asked which, as multiple questions tend to be, are usually self-defeating. C's phrasing, ". . . what's *wrong* with her?", has a relatively high emotional valence, too high, given the level of the counselees' defensiveness.

W: I never think of her having anything wrong—

W responds defensively with denial. She is saying, "The thoughts of her problems are so unbearable, I do not allow myself to think about them."

C: Really, so. . .

H: Well, I can live with Ann's things, none of these things bother us at all.

C does not really buy W's denial.
H denies that the child's physical defects bother him, thus supporting W's previous denials.

W: Yeah.
[Counselees describe the physical progress the child has made.]

C: O.K. Let me try again. What do you understand are Ann's conditions?

W: Well, I understand that, about, well, I didn't quite understand about the lung . . .

C: [Reviews the facts about the case and concludes by stating that, in the final analysis, he is not sure what caused the multiple malformations in the child.]

W: Well, do you think that, since it was twins, maybe my body couldn't give enough to both of them, so it gave a little to one and a lot to the other.

C: No, no, that doesn't happen. I don't think that happened.

W: Oh. Well, what about, they weren't side by side, they were one on top of another. That's why they didn't know it was twins.

C: [Kindly discounts these postconceptual events and says] It sounds like, to me, that in your mind you have gone over . . .

W: (Simultaneously) Yeah, oh yeah (laughs nervously).

C: —and over and over what went on in that pregnancy and you've been asking yourself, "Is there anything I could have done differently?"

H: (Interrupts) I, next time if we do have another one, she probably won't do nothing wrong (laughs nervously).

W: (Laughs nervously) I was sick . . . (barely audible).

W agrees with H.
The couple presents a united front in resisting C's attempt to deal with the emotional impact of their child's disorder. C is saying, "I am going to try again to get through to you." This is the same question asked above, but, here it is simple, direct, and facilitative.
W begins to respond to C's question, becomes anxious and pulls back by switching the focus of the discussion.
C is derailed by W's response. The degree to which C expresses interest in and responds to evasions of his questions will encourage or discourage more such evasions. It is doubtful how helpful a content reply would be at this point.
W is struggling not only to make sense out of what has happened to her, but to find some reason why she wasn't responsible, that is, she is feeling guilty.

As C attempts to correct the misconception, note that he unwittingly may also be conveying a message that W may be responsible for the child's defects. "Well, if that wasn't it, then I must be responsible, but let me try this one, . . ."

C picks up on the fact that, despite their denials, the couple has been ruminating on Ann's condition. He begins to deal with their guilt feelings. As he speaks, W and later H attempt to block out the painful thoughts that they have been denying, but which C now makes explicit.
This is not agreement. It is an attempt to block out what C is saying.

H hides his own feeling of guilt by blaming W for Ann's condition. He disguises the blame by making his comment sound humorous.
This poignant comment occurs so quickly it is almost lost in the intensity of the moment. On some level, W has

C: Well, look. We see a lot of couples just like you with babies born with multiple defects, and I believe it's normal in a lot of women, and fathers too, to ask questions like this. We say it's a feeling of guilt. That's how we describe it, that maybe if you would have done things differently, things would have turned out all right. But I want to assure you that there is nothing you could have done—

H: (Simultaneously) Yeah. Yeah. I don't feel that way about it.

C: —to have changed this.

W: Well. I don't know. I keep saying that I shouldn't have taken those pills.

C: Sure, you feel responsible in some ways. But there's nothing to suggest that you could have changed the outcome of this.

heard H's blame statement and, in a feeble way, she attempts to defend herself.

C continues. His strategy here is to break through their denial system. He does so by labeling their feelings for them. Until this point he has been very tuned in to the counselees. They, in turn, have slowly begun to expose themselves to him. He then begins to reassure them about their feelings (i.e., he does not accept their feelings). H immediately pulls back and again denies that he feels guilty.

H first blocks out C's statement and then states, "I don't feel guilty."

W does not respond to C's reassurance. She appears to be addressing both H and C here. To the former she is saying, "Maybe you don't feel guilty but I do." To C she is saying, "I do not agree with you that there was nothing I could have done. I could have not taken those pills." She has apparently not been reassured by C.

The choreography of this segment of the counseling session may be outlined somewhat as follows: C first attempts to ascertain the counselees' future reproductive plans. He exposes a tender area of possible unresolved feelings and marital conflict; H's desire to delay further reproduction suggests to C that the couple has not completed working through painful feelings connected with the birth of the defective child. Next, he attempts to help the counselees verbalize their feelings. The latter resist this tactic. C then moves to undermine their rationalization by directing their attention to the most obvious fact (and thus the most difficult one to deny), their child's defects. However, H and W continue to resist and again they form a wall against the counselor. C persists and reopens the question of how the counselees feel about the defects. This time, he directs his remarks to W, sensing that her defenses may not be as strong as H's. His tactic is to break up their coalition. Again W resists, this time by shifting the focus of C's attention to another subject. She succeeds in doing this temporarily. C then begins to lay out W's unspoken thoughts and, as he does, her anxiety level rises rapidly. She gives H verbal and, presumably, nonverbal messages that she can no longer play the game of, "Let's pretend that everything's O.K." H is angered at W for placing him in a more vulnerable position by lowering her defenses. He attacks her and blames her for causing the child's defects. This isolates W and permits her to ally herself with C, and by so doing, allows her to express her own sense of guilt. C does not go back to the issue of H blaming W for what has happened.

C's strategy is not without its risks. It seems to have worked at least partially for W, but not for H. His interventions have tended to highlight the points of discord between them, thus possibly exacerbating whatever marital dysfunctions already exist. In family therapy, this is a commonly used tactic to break down dysfunctional ways of relating so that more adaptive ones can be established. In working with such families, however, the counselor generally maintains a relatively longer working relationship than that of the genetic counseling situation.

The next transcript deals with a couple in their early 30s with personality styles somewhat similar to the previous couple. They have one living child, 3 years old, with a shunted hydrocephalus. The condition became evident shortly after the child's birth and now the couple has been thinking of having another child. The following exchange occurred within the first minutes of the session:

C: I wonder what it is you tell your-self about Marty's condition?

This is a simple facilitative question for eliciting feelings.

W: [She talks around the question and finally says that she had a prolonged labor which ended in a caesarian section.]

C: Do you think that's why Marty had the hydrocephalus?

C's question informs W that he recognizes that she feels guilty.

W: Yes, I guess I do. Also I took aspirin during the pregnancy.

Her responibility and guilt quickly emerge in response to C's empathic attention.

C: So in some ways you hold yourself reponsible for the fact that Marty was born with a hydrocephalus.

C reflects back W's sense of responsibility. He does not use the word, "guilt" to provide W the space to label her feelings that way if she so chooses.

W: Yes, I know it's silly, but I do.

C: So you know that those things had no connection with the hydro-cephalus, yet on another level you still hold yourself responsible. I wonder if you know that most couples in your situation do what

C informs the counselees that it is O.K. to feel the way they do. It is normal, others in the same position feel the same way. (It may be surprising, but some couples do not know that their experience has some universality.)

you are doing, in that they wonder
whether or not, if they had done
something different, things would
have turned out differently?
W: Yeah. I suppose I know but it
still feels that way.
C: Sure, sure it does. You know there   C accepts W's feelings and admits his
is really nothing I can say that will   own inability to alter them. This turns
or can change those feelings.   out to be a crucial intervention.
H: At first, I blamed myself . . .   C's acceptance of W's feelings allows
[He goes on to describe his initial   H to relieve himself of his own sense of
reactions and how he finally made   responsibility. He blurts out this state-
his peace with his feelings.]   ment as if he has long needed to make
                                           a public confession. This may have been
                                           difficult for him to say. C has created a
                                           safe environment in which H can take
                                           the risk of sharing his feelings.
C: So both of you, in your own ways,   A nonjudgemental reflecting back of what
have felt some responsibility for   the counselees have said.
Marty's condition.
W: Yes. It's better now for both of us,
but every once in a while I think
about it.
C: Uh, huh. I suppose it is difficult to   Rather than attempt to reassure, C re-
accept the fact that there was   flects back how difficult it is to accept
nothing you might have done to   one's impotency and helplessness to con-
change what was going to happen.   trol one's life. This is a statement of
                                           acceptance of their feelings.

In contrast to the session of the first transcript, the one above appears
to be less structured. C has less of a personal agenda. His opening query
is open-ended and allows the counselees to make a choice as to the direction in which they wish the session to go, into content matters or into
feelings. W's response reveals that she harbors unresolved feelings of
responsibility for her child's defects. C's empathic responses allow both
counselees to express their feelings. At each point, he simply accepts their
feelings and does not attempt to alter, reassure or otherwise convey the
message that their feelings are not legitimate. Also, he has planted important ideas which the counselees may use constructively as they continue to work-through their feelings.

In the next transcript a couple with a 5-year old child with a split hand
and foot deformity is being counseled. The couple is in their mid-20s. W
was pregnant when the couple initiated the request for genetic counseling, but underwent a therapeutic abortion several days prior to the counseling itself. This was the third therapeutic abortion in as many years.
The transcript begins about 5 minutes into the session; the abortion is
under discussion.

C: This seems to be doing terrible things to your head.

W: Uh, huh. I feel like a murderer, you know (her eyes well up). . . . I'd like to hear more about what's in that folder there (points to hospital record).

Her feelings begin to overwhelm her and she defends herself by switching the focus to another thought.

C: I can appreciate that you're anxious to get into this, but I'm wondering if you could for a moment stick with that feeling, of feeling like a. . . .

Rather than deal with content here, C brings W back to the earlier distressing thought.

W: Oh, yeah. I do, I really do. (She begins to cry.) What can I say, it's not like you've had a miscarriage. That's not your fault. But, you know I guess it's my family background. I've always been raised religiously and everything. I feel like,. in God's eyes, He really looks down on me. And it's not just God, myself.

She has betrayed the ideals by which she has been raised.

C: It sounds to me that you're disappointed in what you've done.

W: You should have heard the expression in their voices when I told them I had three abortions, especially Dr. E's expression was like— (she breaks off).

C: What was it that you heard in his voice?

W: Kind of anger, kind of disgust.

W may be projecting here, but it is conceivable that Dr. E was actually disgusted with her. C might have said "It sounds like that might be the way *you* feel about yourself."

C: I can see how much this hurts you and I can see how harshly you've already judged yourself. It seems to me that, as you look back at the decisions you've made, they haven't made you feel very good about yourself. I'm wondering what thoughts you've given to steps that would prevent that from happening again?

C is conveying the message that the past cannot be undone, nevertheless, it need not be repeated. Another way C might have proceeded to explore the couple's plans for the future would have been to ask, "I'm wondering, as you look back at your past decisions, what is it that you would change if you could?"

In contrast to the situations discussed in previous transcripts, the couple in the transcript above had a choice with respect to their behavior and are more directly responsible for their present situation and psychological state. C does not sit in judgment. He accepts W's feelings and attempts to reframe her guilt in a way so that it can be used as a motivator for different responses in the future.

The couple in the following transcript is receiving counseling for neural tube defects following the neonatal death of a child with hydrocephalus the previous year. Both counselees appear to be of average intelligence. W is currently pregnant. At the point at which the transcript begins, the session is nearing its end. C has explained in some detail the various causes of hydrocephalus and their modes of inheritance. Most of his transactions have been with H; W has been minimally involved. Just prior to the beginning of the transcript, H has asked a series of questions which suggest that he has guilt feelings about the child and that he has not entirely been following all the content material that C has provided. C has just finished discussing the genetic basis of neural tube defects, at which point, C2, a female counselor present in the session, turns to W and inquires:

C2: Do you understand that, Mrs. Baker?

> To this point the session has virtually been a dialogue between C and H. C2 attempts to involve W.

W: I don't know (sighs).

> W sounds overwhelmed, helpless and childlike. For most of the session, she has been virtually ignored by the men. Feeling discounted and not being able to find a role for herself in the session, she remains silent.

C2: It is kind of complicated.

> This is an empathic response to W which might have led to an expression of the issues on W's mind.

C: [Shifts gears at this point and obtains a detailed family history.]

> C interrupts C2's work with W and reasserts direction of the session. C may be responding to something nonverbal about W that may make him want to minimize her involvement in the session and/or he feels that he cannot handle her needs.

W: Doesn't it look awful when you start taking histories of people? I hate it.

> She feels shame and wants C's approval. She is asking, "Am I awful?" She has a low sense of self-esteem.

C2: You know that every family has something—

> C2 attempts to reassure W.

W: (Interrupts) *His* doesn't, it's just mine.

> Presumably she has experienced or felt blame in the past and is smarting. Like H, W also feels responsible for the birth of the defective child. She does not appear to be reassured.

C: We'll see. We'll see. How was that pregnancy with this baby, the one that died?

C does not respond to W's feelings.

W: Well, yeah, it was crummy (her voice shakes), the whole thing was crummy. [She goes on to describe her nausea and discomfort and the fact that she had a cold about 3–4 months into the pregnancy.]

C: Let me reassure you that 3–4 months is already too late in the pregnancy to produce this type of damage in the fetus.

C attempts to reassure W that she is not responsible for her baby's defects. Again, he does not respond to W's feelings.

W: Could I ask something right now?

W does not respond to C's reassurance suggesting that its meaning has failed to hit home. C and W are not making contact. She experiences herself as powerless and thus must ask permission of C to interrupt.

C: Anytime.

W: I don't know anything about it, but just the way I feel about it. She was *so* bad, couldn't that have, wouldn't that mean that from the very beginning it happened to be that severe, I mean—

W is clearly informing C that her cognitive understanding is more affective rather than a factual one. She then begins to share her understanding of the child's defects in the context of asking a question presumably about her responsibility for "causing" the defects during the pregnancy. She is asking for reassurance that she didn't cause the defect by her behavior during the pregnancy.

C: (Interrupts) You mean from the very beginning? From conception? [C again explains the genetic origins of the defect.]

C responds to the content of W's aborted question. Since she has already stated that facts won't cut much ice with her, C's approach is likely to be futile. In fact, he sounds frustrated, as he is repeating explanations provided earlier in the session. A possibly more productive statement might have been, "It seems to me that in some way you hold yourself responsible for your child's defects."

W: I just don't want to think that anything I did hurt that baby. That really upsets me. I could just—

Here is an opportunity for C to make a statement along the lines: "Of course that would be upsetting. I'm wondering if that's what you do think nonetheless?"

C: (Interrupts) I don't think so too. And furthermore, the search for what you may have done or not done is absolutely useless be-

C recognizes that W is feeling responsible for the defects, yet he does not acknowledge or respond to W's feelings. Because this has been omitted, his re-cause. . . . [He goes on to explain how environmental agents and pollutants might cause birth defects.]

assurance at this point is not likely to be heard.

W does not respond to C's statement.

C: [Goes on to explain ultrasound and amniocentesis procedures in connection with alpha-fetoprotein determination.]

W: Do most people go ahead and have this in our situation?

W is asking for C's advice as to whether or not to have the amniocentesis. She is still in role as a child.

C: (Cautiously) Do most people? I can't answer. What do you mean by "most?" By far the largest group of couples who come for amniocentesis are women of age 35 or above. [He distinguishes between most women and most women referred to the clinic specifically for the procedure.]

Again, C responds to the content of W's question. He supplies her with information which is irrelevant to her question. (For an alternative response, see p. 88.) This particular couple may have considerable difficulty in reaching important decisions; W's sense of helplessness, their unresolved feelings of guilt, they are blaming one another (see W's statement above, "His doesn't, it's just mine.") and a lack of mutual support (note how conspicuously absent H has been during these several transactions between C and W) all are indicators of the need for the counselor to focus more on interpersonal issues if C wants the factual material to be heard. One might speculate that W's question relates to what C had said earlier regarding the uselessness of trying to determine the cause of the child's defects.

W: Do these things happen just because, I mean, for no reason?

In context here, it has no obvious relationship to what C has just told her. W and C are not together; therefore, their statements and questions are out of touch. W's question reveals something about the way she views the world. She tends to see events as governed by chance and thus rational decision making may be out of her domain of planning.

C: There's nothing that has no reason. . . .

C sounds incredulous. His tone conveys the metamessage, "How could you ask such a silly question?" His reply is as characterological for him as W's question was for her. C sees the world as governed by principles of causality. He is informing W that, "You and I do not think alike."

W: (Simultaneously) No, I mean. . . .

W tries to recoup and clarify what it is that she is asking. She may have made a fool of herself in C's eyes and may be feeling humiliated. She wants to please C, so she will back off from interrupting him.

C: [Explains genetic mechanisms again.]

C is saying, "See, all things have causes."

W: But you would advise, would you. . . .

C: (Simultaneously) Well—

W: —to have it?

C: I, that's not my decision to make. All I can tell you—

W: Well—

C: —what the procedure is and what the risks are—

W: (Interrupts) Yeah, but if it were your sister sitting there, and she, I mean, if, I don't—

C: (Interrupts) I wouldn't be able to advise my sister on what to do.

W has the expectation that C will take charge and tell her what to do. C has not to this point dispelled this belief. From W's viewpoint, C has held out a carrot and now he is pulling it away. She must end up disappointed and feeling rejected. One thing C might do at this point is to reflect back that she wants him to make a decision for her and he will not do that even if that means that he will disappoint her. Another approach is to reflect back that perhaps W is disappointed in him for not advising her straightaway and perhaps he has been remiss for not having made his own (nondirective) position clearer to her. By assuming his share of the responsibility of what has not occurred in the session, C may relieve W of the full burden of responsibility that there is something wrong or reprehensible about herself that leads to such rejection from authority figures.

C2: [Intervenes and explains the nondirective stance the counselor is taking.] So it is impossible for us to advise you whether to have the procedure or not.

W: I'm just afraid of losing the baby.

W sounds calm here. She has been

C: From the tap? That I can reassure you. . . . [He talks about the low risks involved.]

treated like an adult and now she can open up and express her fear clearly and succinctly.

C attempts to provide W with facts that he thinks will reduce her fear. What *she* wants is for him to say, "I can understand your fear. Most women who have this procedure have some fears about it (i.e., your fears are not abnormal)."

W: The test isn't painful, is it?

Perhaps, then she might be more receptive to the facts he would like to convey. When a fear or concern has been reassured it is generally followed by some release of affect or other signs indicating that some inner change has occurred. A lack of such signs suggests that the fear or concern has been untouched. W does not respond to C's reassurance, she expresses another concern.

C: [Draws comparison to drawing blood sample and how different people respond.] There's some people who'll say it is not painful and there are other people who will faint—

W is too suggestible for examples of this kind.

W: (Interrupts) Oh, God, I'd be fainting all the time, I think (laughs).

In contrast to W's defensively helpless stance earlier, here she seems able to laugh at herself.

C: [Describes some of the facts about amniocentesis.]

W: I guess we know already, I won't decide anything. (Her voice is childlike.)

Touché.

The most conspicuous aspect of the previous transcript is the degree to which the male counselor and the counselees fail to make contact with each other. This is largely due to the personality differences between C and W, although marital difficulties between H and W may also contribute. Each expects the other to respond and to understand them in terms of their own frame of reference, never stopping to consider that the other person has a different way of understanding the world.

The respective ways of relating to the world of C and of W are almost diametrically opposite. C tends to understand the world in a technical, detailed manner, whereas, W's approach is intuitive and impressionistic. Their two styles are complementary. In the psychological-psychiatric literature, their interactions have frequently been discussed under the heading of the obsessive-hysteric relationship (Barnett, 1971; MacKinnon & Michels, 1971).[4]

Although genetic counseling is not considered to be a form of psychotherapy, psychotherapeutic consequences may nonetheless ensue. For example, C2's timely intervention in which she explains why the counselors will not make decisions for H and W has a profound effect on W's subsequent behavior in the session. W becomes less defensive. She expresses her concerns more clearly and openly, her ability to manage her anxiety increases, and she begins to see her own behavior in a more realistic light. These are the very kinds of changes one sees during the course of a therapeutic session.

The previous transcript also illustrates how important it is to attend to the psychodynamics of the counseling and how failing to do so may interfere with the provision of information and with the counselees' ability to reach personally relevant decisions. One sometimes hears the argument, "There just isn't enough time to deal with the psychological problems we see in genetic counseling." The argument is specious. One properly

---

[4] In general, obsessives and hysterics tend to see in each other the characteristics which they sense are lacking in themselves. Thus, they are often attracted to one another and marry. The hysteric sees the obsessive as stable, organized, self-controlled, and profound whereas the latter sees the former as warm, insightful, vivacious, and loving. The initial idealizations of the outward aspects of the other often leads to disappointment and conflict in such relationships; neither wants to see the neediness motivating the other's behavior.

Although both types of personality are found in the two sexes, in Western societies the role expectations of males and females are frequently shaped in the direction of obsessive and hysteric traits respectively. Thus, difficulties between obsessives and hysterics generally interface with sexist issues.

In the counseling situation, the female hysteric's style of trying to obtain emotional support may be experienced by the male obsessive counselor as overly demanding, which, in turn, may generate feelings of wanting to distance and extricate himself. This he generally does by using his intellectuality and other characterological responses. She, on her side, may experience such behavior as disinterest or as rejection. At worst, she may feel punished.

In the physician–patient interaction, the female hysteric often:

> presents herself as helpless and dependent, relying on the . . . responses of the physician in order to guide her every action. [She views him] . . . as magically omnipotent and capable of solving . . . her problems in some mysterious fashion. [He] . . . is expected to take care of [her] and assume all responsibility . . . as though her own efforts did not count. This leads to major countertransference problems in the doctor who enjoys the opportunity to enter an omnipotent alliance [MacKinnon & Michels, 1971].

Of course, in the genetic counseling situation, the fostering of such relationships would be antithetical to the development of the autonomous, self-directed thinking needed to control one's life and make one's own decisions.

timed intervention, so-to-speak empathically on the mark, may actually avoid needless explanations and diversions and may facilitate the transmission of factual material. For the same investment of time in the face-to-face encounter with the counselees, the genetic counselor could be considerably more effective in accomplishing the tasks of genetic counseling by dealing directly with psychological issues. At the same time, the counselor may have a therapeutic influence on the counselees, individually and as a couple.

Summary Phase

As the session draws to a close, it is often a good idea to review briefly the salient points that have been discussed. The counselors may ask the counselees what they perceived the highlights of the session to be, and then they might provide their own perceptions and integrative statements. An alternative approach is for the counselor to take the lead in summarizing the major issues discussed and then to ask the counselees if they perceived any points that might have been missed. The task of this phase is to unify and integrate the various themes raised during the course of the counseling. This provides an opportunity for the counselor to reinforce earlier interpretations. For example, earlier in a session with a couple with obvious marital difficulties, the counselor may have commented that they seemed to have strongly different feelings about several major issues in their relationship. In the summary phase, this might be pointed out again and the question advanced as to what thoughts they have given to seeking help to work out their differences. Also, this phase of the counseling session would be the appropriate point to restate the genetic risk and other major medical facts without introducing new data. Last, the counselor may want to differentiate between the issues on which the counselees have reached closure and those on which they have not. For example, if a decision concerning a medical procedure or reproduction has been reached in the session, it would be worthwhile for the counselor to state his or her understanding of the decision and to check out with the counselees if their understanding is the same. Similarly, if an issue was raised concerning which no decision was made, this too should be pointed out.

THE FOLLOW-UP

A follow-up interview with the counselees is a desirable procedure. It provides an opportunity to determine the extent to which they have integrated the material discussed during the previous counseling. Also, it may allow the counselees to reassess decisions and actions from a different time frame. With distance, the person may see the same facts from a new vantage point. This may allow a new and higher order of integration than that achieved earlier.

The follow-up session might be used by the counselor to sample the counselees' memory for factual details and to repeat previously provided information. The term "reinforcement" is generally employed in the literature to describe such repetitions. What may be reinforced in addition to the counselees' factual understanding is unclear. If previously provided information has been grossly distorted, an attempt to correct the situation should be made. However, it may be as important for the counselor to explore the issues possibly contributing to the counselees' misperceptions. If the original or similar conditions continue to exist which promoted the original misperceptions, it is likely that further misperceptions will occur.

The follow-up may also give the counselors an opportunity to evaluate the effect of their work with the counselees. What decisions were made as a consequence of the counseling? What effect did the counseling have on the counselees' relationship? If, for example, a separation or divorce occurred following the counseling session, could this have been foretold from an analysis of a recording or transcript of the session?

The decisions taken following the counseling session may have had serious repercussions for the family; financial, marital, psychological, and otherwise. The follow-up session should provide for an exploration of the issues raised as a consequence of the counseling.

Lastly, an opportunity is needed for the counselees to provide the counselor with feedback. What was it that helped them? What did not? What might the counselor have done differently from their vantage point? The follow-up is a good place for the counselees to express gratitude and/or resentments that circumstances did not permit earlier.

In scheduling follow-up sessions, a balance is needed between intruding too early and contacting the counselees too long after the counseling for maximum effectiveness. There are no simple rules. Each case will need an individual approach. Following the elective abortion of a Down's fetus detected as a result of amniocentesis, a follow-up telephone call at about 2 weeks after the abortion seems a reasonable length of time to wait. During the call, an invitation can be extended to meet face-to-face in about another 2–3 weeks or earlier, if the counselees feel ready to do so. After such a follow-up interview, another telephone call might be made about 4–6 weeks later. In each case, the counselees should be apprised in advance of the counselor's intention to call them to make arrangements for further contact. This reduces the surprise element and tends to minimize possible anxiety related to further contacts with the clinic.

In many instances, a follow-up session in the counselees' home or in a place other than the one in which the original counseling took place would be most desirable. The original site may have a high emotional valence that may interfere with the assessment of the consequences of the counseling.

Epilogue

Each counseling session generally has its own inner logic and unity. Examination of transcripts of genetic counseling sessions suggests that a stepwise progression occurs in the session which, in outline, recapitulates the major tasks along the course of individual human development. Adequate resolution of the tasks of one stage provides the seedbed for the resolution of issues of subsequent stages. In the initial phases of the genetic counseling session, just as in the early months of human life, the key issue is the establishment of mutual trust. Erikson (1963) writes "that the amount of trust derived from earliest infantile experience does not seem to depend on absolute quantities of food or demonstrations of love, but rather on the quality of the maternal relationship [p. 249]." Similarly, in genetic counseling it is probably not the amount of information or number of reassurances provided but rather the *quality* of the counselor–counselee relationship which determines the establishment of mutual trust. Failures in this area will interfere with the accomplishment of later tasks in the session.

In the next stage of the counseling, the major task is facilitating the development of a sense of autonomy. Overprotectiveness, reassurances, and the need to display one's own competence, knowledge, and power on the part of the professional impede the development of autonomy in the counselees, which, in turn, undermines the development of initiative to plan and undertake actions on one's own behalf. In his discussion of the early growth of competence in the child, White (1972) writes:

> The most important way in which parents can support a child's initiative is to feel and communicate *respect*. This . . . means to notice and appreciate the child's ability, as shown in his manifestations of competence . . . Respect dwindles, . . . if the parent starts congratulating himself on having brought the child up well, displacing the credit to himself [p. 219].

There is much in the child development literature for genetic counselors to ponder; good counseling is comparable to good parenting.

Underlying genetic counseling is an issue which, in the normal sequence of human development, occurs in adulthood. Erikson (1963) refers to it as the issue of generativity, "the concern in establishing and guiding the next generation [p. 267]." This is stage VII in the "Eight Ages of Man." Frustration of this stage of development has important psychosocial consequences that Erikson summarizes as a pervading sense of personal stagnation and impoverishment. It is the threat to the successful accomplishment of this life stage that brings many individuals and couples to the genetic counselor in the first place. How the counselor helps the counselees deal with the issue of generativity must have long-range effects on their further psychosocial development and on the degree to which they achieve ego integration and give their lives a sense of meaning. Viewed in this context, genetic counseling is as salient a human interaction as any other psychologically oriented counseling activity.

References

Angyl, A. *Neurosis and treatment: A holistic theory.* New York: J. Wiley and Sons, 1965.

Barnett, J. Narcissism and dependency in the obsessional-hysteric marriage. *Family Process,* 1971, *10,* 75–83.

Berne, E. *Games people play.* New York: W. W. Norton and Co., 1964.

Erikson, E. H. *Childhood and society.* New York: W. W. Norton and Co., 1963.

MacKinnon, R. A. & Michels, R. *The psychiatric interview in clinical practice.* Philadelphia: W. B. Saunders Co., 1971.

Rotter, J. B. Generalized expectancies for internal versus external control of reinforcement. *Psychological Monographs,* 1966, *80*(1), Whole No. 609.

Salzman, L. *The obsessive personality.* New York: Jason Aronson, 1973.

Shapiro, D. *Neurotic styles.* New York: Basic Books, 1965.

White, R. W. *The enterprise of living.* New York: Holt, Rinehart and Winston, 1972.

Amniocentesis Counseling 6

Rose Grobstein

One of the most important advances of recent years is the development of transabdominal amniocentesis. This procedure has made possible the prenatal diagnosis of the chromosomal disorders and an ever-growing list of genetic diseases. With the sanction of the relevant medical societies, mid-trimester amniocentesis has been characterized as a "highly accurate and safe procedure that does not significantly increase the risk of fetal loss or injury [NICHD Study Group, 1976]." Information on the procedure has been disseminated by professional journals, lay magazines, and the mass media. As a consequence, an increasing number of women are requesting amniocentesis and an increasing number of obstetricians are referring women, especially those 35 years of age and over, to prenatal diagnostic centers to have the procedure done. Many obstetricians do not perform the procedure themselves and, since the amniotic fluid requires skilled handling, individuals are frequently referred to genetic counseling clinics in medical centers. In such clinics, the prospective parents are often counseled; the procedure and related technical issues are explained, and the risks to both mother and fetus are discussed. In short, an attempt is made to obtain an "informed consent."

Although these explanations of the procedures and risks are absolutely necessary, it needs to be questioned whether this alone constitutes an adequate basis for obtaining truly "informed consent." It is my contention that the counselor has a much greater responsibility than merely giving information regarding the risks of the procedure. This is only a first step. Also involved are a series of complex decision-making components, a

107

GENETIC COUNSELING
Psychological Dimensions

discussion of which is a central aspect of any preamniocentesis counseling aimed at obtaining an "informed consent" for the procedure. This point does not appear to be widely appreciated by many referring physicians as many couples are surprised that they are expected to attend a counseling session prior to having the procedure and most (some) are not prepared for the psychosocial concomitants of what is initially presented to them as a "simple" medical procedure.

In the discussion which follows, I plan to discuss the decision-making components associated with the amniocentesis procedure. I will limit the discussion to the group of couples referred to the genetic counselor for reasons of maternal age. Couples who are referred for counseling because of the possibility or presence of a known X-linked, recessive or dominant disorder constitute a different population and will not be considered here.

The key decision-making points that need to be considered in amniocentesis counseling may be conceptualized as questions, which from the couple's point of view are as follows:

1. Should we have the procedure?
2. If we do have the procedure and the results show the presence of a child with abnormal chromosomes, what is to be done?
3. What impact will a second trimester abortion have?
4. Should we try to have another pregnancy after the abortion? When? What will our anxiety be like during another waiting period?

In deciding whether or not to have the procedure, most couples take several factors into account. First, there is a baseline of information regarding amniocentesis gleaned from discussion with the referring physician, newspaper and magazine articles, radio and television programs, and, increasingly, from others who have had the procedure themselves. This baseline knowledge may be, but often is not, very accurate; nevertheless, it is of a nature sufficient to motivate the couple to come in for the counseling. Presumably, most of such couples are already predisposed to having the procedure, else they would not have proceeded this far.

There are some couples who come in for counseling solely at the behest of (or to please) their physician and with little obvious intrinsic motivation. They are often highly suggestible, and care needs to be taken by the counselor to avoid being parental and directive. The full implications of going ahead with the procedure and the possible decisions they may have to face should a fetus with a chromosomal disorder be detected, needs to be communicated to all couples, but in particular to poorly motivated ones before they arrive at a decision to have or to decline the procedure.

One of the major tasks of the counselor early on in amniocentesis counseling is to ascertain the counselees' level of understanding of the procedure. Hopefully, a decision to have or not to have the procedure is based on correct, undistorted information. The potential for later disappointment is probably heightened if the decision for or against the procedure is based on misinformation.

A second factor taken into account is the perceived increased risk for a child with Down's Syndrome. Presumably, a couple who perceives this risk as being substantially higher than that of the procedure itself will be biased toward having the procedure. The meaning of the risk needs to be explored with the couple. To obtain true "informed consent" the counselor may need to raise several issues. For example, for many couples, the absolute risk for a Down's syndrome fetus is less than 1%. Is it sensible to go through the amniocentesis procedure (and its concomitant expense) when the risk is of that low magnitude? Also, the counselor needs to point out that even though the procedure is carried out and a report of normal chromosomes is made, it does not provide the couple with assurance that the child will be physically and mentally normal. Few couples know that the general population risk of having a child with a major birth defect is somewhere between 3 and 5% and that a small fraction of these defects are detectable through amniocentesis, albeit those which are detectable often have major phenotypic consequences.

With couples who consider their risk for a Down's syndrome child too low to warrant having the procedure, counselors may want to help the couple look at the possible impact on the entire family of having a child with a chromosomal defect (Schild, 1977). They might ask whether or not they have given any thought to that possibility, whether or not they personally know couples with a Down's syndrome child and how they were affected, and so on. Also, they might ask them to consider what the possible burdens, financial, and psychological might be of having such a child. How will it affect their life style and what consequences might it have for each member of the family, adults and children alike.

Another factor influencing whether or not the couple proceeds with the procedure is their attitude toward abortion. Many couples oppose abortion for religious and other reasons, and sometimes decline the procedure because they are confident that even if they knew that the fetus had an abnormality, they would not abort it. Some couples who also oppose abortion, nevertheless decide to go ahead with the amniocentesis. It would be beyond the scope of this chapter to go into the various reasons why this occurs. Suffice it to say that for some couples the threat of a deformed or defective child is so strong that long-held beliefs and values are subordinated to the desire for a healthy infant.

It is important for the counselor to ascertain whether both spouses are in accord with respect to wanting the amniocentesis procedure and having an abortion should a chromosome disorder be detected. Not infrequently, a husband might say that since the wife is having the procedure, it is really her decision to make. A variant of this occurs when the husband expresses the viewpoint that since his wife is carrying the baby, it is up to her whether or not to have an abortion. Rationally, he might be right, but life and relationships do not work that way. The counselor should help the husband express his feelings about the amniocentesis, so that both mates know where the other stands. (With respect to within-couple differences regarding abortion, see the comments that follow.)

Prior to undergoing the amniocentesis procedure, the couple should understand that there will be a waiting period of several weeks before the results of the chromosomal analysis are known. This period is one filled with anxiety and may be particularly difficult for the women.

I recall phoning a family to tell them of the normal results of the chromosome study. The woman answered the phone, and, after I had identified myself, I added that the child she was carrying had normal chromosomes. She immediately starting crying and handed the phone to her husband. He explained that she had been anxiously awaiting my call, and that the relief was overwhelming. Imagine the anxiety she had been experiencing!

Some couples begin telephoning the clinic several days before the time the results were "promised" to them in the hope of obtaining advance information. It is clear that many couples who have the procedure are keenly aware of the fact that they are waiting with anticipation and anxiety. Frequently, when calling couples to give them the "good news," one can hear the deep sigh of relief as the person on the other end of the line resumes breathing after literally holding their breath out of anxiety and fear of learning that their baby is "defective."

Should the couple decide to have the amniocentesis, a major question to explore is what will they do should the results show a child with abnormal chromosomes? Most couples answer that they will have an abortion. But, they may not have considered that the abortion will be done at 18 to 20 weeks of pregnancy and that frequently the woman has already felt "quickening." Also, they may not know that a second trimester abortion means experiencing a shortened labor and accepting the termination of the pregnancy. There are also certain medical risks involved with such abortion, such as chills, fever, hemorrhage, uterine rupture, or infection which need to be discussed. More than 95% of the counseled couples decide to have amniocentesis after considering all these points. The overriding consideration seems to be the desire to avoid having a mentally defective child. It needs to be remembered that the couple is not imminently faced with the necessity of undergoing an abortion and thus the discussion of these matters may proceed smoothly and rationally. Not infrequently, the subject of abortion is so threatening or emotionally laden that evidence of past unresolved conflicts, current marital difficulties, and the like may emerge. The counselor needs to be able to help the couple deal with these charged issues. Considerable evidence suggests that persons who have anticipated future trauma seem to be able to deal with it more effectively than those who have not done anticipatory work.

For the 96.5% of couples who hear the comforting words, "Your child has normal chromosomes," the decision making in this area ends. However, for the 3.5% who are asked to return to the genetic counseling clinic to discuss their child's abnormal chromosomes, the decision making and concerns continue. This is the time when the counselor must be exquisitely sensitive to the couples' responses to this information. In a very short period of time the counselor must help the couple come to a decision about the pregnancy. If it has not already begun, anticipatory grief has undoubtedly started with the counselor's phone call. It may be grieving for the loss of the "perfect child" or it may be grieving for the actual loss of the child. Hopefully, the couple has discussed their feelings and the possible course of action they will take during the waiting period.[1] Most couples, however, feel that it will not happen to them and they have a variety of rationalizations, ranging from the good state of their own health to the fact that an aunt had three perfectly healthy children after age 38.

Regardless of previous discussions, the reality of carrying a defective child is a great shock. The couple experiences all the feelings of disbelief, anger, depression, and guilt that accompany the birth of a child with a defect. The counselor needs to help the parents with these feelings while simultaneously helping them to come to a decision whether or not to abort. Usually, because of statutory requirements, time is critical, and a great deal of emotional support needs to be given during this period. Often, the couple may need more than one counseling session in order to come to terms with their decision. It is extremely important that the couple arrive at the decision jointly. No counselor should ignore the partner's statement that it is "her decision." "She is carrying the baby and has to go through the abortion." Both must accept the responsibility for the decision made so that later feelings of guilt and recriminations are not used to increase marital discord. It took two to create the child. It should take two to decide to terminate the pregnancy or to raise the child.

When a couple has decided on abortion, the anguish and indecision

[1] In the course of counseling, counselees should be encouraged to discuss these matters during the later waiting period with due recognition that it is not a pleasant topic or an easy one on which to focus.

is not over. I have found that talking with them during the abortion procedure has been experienced by the couple as extremely supportive. The need for them to feel that their decision is an acceptable one is great and the counselor's visits during the abortion procedure are viewed as an affirmation that the decision made was the right one for the couple concerned.

After the abortion supportive counseling is needed (Blumberg, Golbus, & Hanson, 1975). The feelings of guilt and inadequacy with resulting depression all need time for resolution. Couples need to know that mourning is a normal process following an abortion. They have, indeed, lost a child. Frequently the woman, in particular, has the task of resolving her feelings of being the "cause" of the family's anguish and of the "death" of the child.

I would like to tell you about the S family. Mr. and Mrs. S., ages 38 and 36, had been married for 10 years. They had postponed childbearing until their business was successful since it necessitated that both of them work very hard to accomplish this. It was obvious that this was a couple who had planned their lives carefully and everything had fallen into its expected place.

Both looked upon the amniocentesis as a routine procedure, much as one would view a premarital examination. The amniocentesis, however, revealed that Mrs. S. was carrying a Down's child with a translocation. The first postamniocentesis session was extremely difficult for everyone with both members of the couple crying and being very supportive of each other. The decision to have an abortion was made, and everything went well. However, the fact of the translocation had really not been absorbed. The third session was held after the individual chromosomes of the couple had been studied. The results showed that Mrs. S. was carrying a balanced translocation. This information came as a great shock to both, but, as one might expect, particularly to Mrs. S. She called herself "damaged" and felt that she could never have a child. The husband tried to comfort her, but she was devastated. The counselors spent considerable time talking with the couple. Information was given them regarding the presence of abnormal genes in everyone, and that in their case, it was, perhaps, fortunate that they had postponed child-bearing since the translocation might have appeared at anytime. This, of course, was small comfort to Mrs. S. and finally she accepted a referral to an outside agency for further counseling. Her self-image had, indeed, been damaged, and it was necessary that she receive assistance in reconstructing it.

Once the mourning period is over, the next decision-making point concerns the issue of whether or not to try to have another child and possibly to subject themselves to the above process once again. What will it be like to go through the waiting process again, even though the odds are in their favor? Will they be able to go through another abortion should the results once again be unfavorable? What will it mean to them as a family should they decide not to have another or, perhaps, any children? These are not easy questions to answer, and, frequently, couples will need to explore them with the aid of an appropriate counselor.

It should be abundantly clear that amniocentesis involves considerably more than a simple, ordinary medical procedure. Involved in undertaking the procedure are major psychosocial concomitants which may have important long-range consequences for the couple and their family. Consenting to the procedure without understanding its psychosocial as well as its technical implications is not true informed consent. In my experience, it takes an average of nearly 1 hour of counseling to discuss the main points that need to be covered in preamniocentesis counseling. Community physicians and other referral resources need to be apprised of the importance of referring couples sufficiently ahead of time so that adequate counseling can be provided and so that adequate decision-making time is available to the couple.

References

Blumberg, B. D., Golbus, M. S. & Hanson, K. H. The psychological sequelae of abortion performed for a genetic indication. *American Journal of Obstetrics and Gynecology*, 1975, *122*, 799–808.

NICHD Study Group. Midtrimester amniocentesis for prenatal diagnosis: Safety and accuracy, *Journal of the American Medical Association*, 1976, *236*, 1471–1476.

Schild, S. Social work with genetic problems. *Health and Social Work*, 1977, *2*, 59–77.

Genetic Counseling for Parents of a Baby with Down's Syndrome[1]

7

Ray M. Antley

Following the birth of a child with Down's syndrome (DS), parents often seek genetic counseling for several reasons. They need information to gain some understanding of the disorder as well as to have a basis for making decisions about future courses of action. Also, they have concerns about the validity of the diagnosis, the prognosis, potential interventions, and the recurrence risk. In what follows, I have attempted to present an approach to providing genetic counseling to parents who have recently had a baby with Down's syndrome. In general terms, I view genetic counseling as a form of nonprescriptive counseling that aims to help the counselees make a series of multidimensional, internally oriented, informed decisions. The genetic counselor needs to accomplish several tasks; the counselor must first determine the counselees' resources, their initial values, the extent of their knowledge of general genetics and of their particular situation. The provision of information must be geared to these conditions and aimed at broadening their base of information. This new information base must then be converted into concepts that can be used by the counselees for evaluating their life situation and into potential options or choices for decision-making purposes. The counselor's most important contribution is not in providing information per se, but in helping the counselees develop a way of dealing with new information. Rather than prescribing an arbitrarily determined "right" set of values, the counselor

[1] This work was supported by Genetics Center Grant (PHS GM 21054), National Institutes of Health Grant (HEW MCHS 924), Grants from the Little Red Door, Inc. and the Riley Memorial Association.

115

helps the counselees gain a better understanding of their problem and their perceptions of it.

Structure for Providing Genetic Counseling

The activities in the genetic counseling clinic and the roles of the various members of the clinic staff need to be coordinated to accomplish the goals of genetic counseling with particular awareness of and attention to the emotional responses of the counselees. From the first contact to the completion of counseling each activity should be evaluated for its effectiveness in terms of its immediate effect on the counselee and its contribution towards accomplishing the counseling goals. For example, at the time of the first contact with the clinic, the genetics assistant attempts to convey the message to the counselees that we expect them to be dependable and responsible and that we will be supportive and open to them. To transmit this dual message, we provide a detailed and structured procedure for them to follow; a specific appointment time with a specific doctor is set, a limited set of materials to fill out ahead of time and a map with verbal instructions on how to find the clinic. This information provides some relief for their situational anxiety and also conveys our expectations of them.

First Clinic Visit

The clinic procedure is designed so that the parents of a child with DS are seen once prior to their being given a definite diagnosis. This provides them with time to accept the possibility that something might be awry with their child, thus allowing for grieving to proceed. Also, the counselees have an opportunity to become acquainted with the counselor, the clinic staff, and the clinic milieu before they have to cope with the cytogenetically confirmed diagnosis. In addition, information about the counselees' personalities is obtained during this visit which prepares the professionals for their task of providing genetic education on future occasions. (See Appendix, p. 129)

Finally, the initial visit offers an opportunity for the genetic staff to make direct interventions at a time when the family is often in shock and crisis. The staff is also able, at this time, to work with the private physician in their attempt to provide care and support. I believe that if the geneticist and the staff see the patient and the family before the chromosome studies are complete the rapport and credibility established between counselees and professionals tends to be improved. In addition, studies of counselees' knowledge prior to counseling indicate that the counselees' level of knowledge is significantly influenced by their having been to the genetics clinic before the genetic counseling visit (Antley, 1977). The time between the two clinic visits is an active one in which the parents read and learn about the child's potential problem.

In the session, an attempt is made to answer questions without getting into long, detailed explanations. Issues are dealt with sufficiently so as to answer the questions the counselees have. If appropriate, the parents are given a paperback book about Down's syndrome (Horrobin & Rynders, 1975). Where their questions anticipate the diagnosis, an attempt is made to defer answering them until after the chromosome studies are completed.

The parents usually have questions about the length of time it takes to get the chromosome results or some other issue with relatively low psychological threat. About half or more of the parents will ask if I think the child has Down's syndrome. I give them my opinion in a probabilistic sense. If there is a high probability, I allow that I am not always correct. Sometimes the counselee will tell me frankly that they believe that I am incorrect. Usually, I reply that I hope they are right and that by the next visit the chromosome study will have provided a definitive answer.

With the exception of the child's intellectual development, parents do not usually raise questions about the major malformations associated with DS. Overall, there is a .8 probability that a child with DS will have at least one major malformation in addition to mental retardation (Roboz & Pitt, 1969). These may include small head size as an adult with mental retardation, bowel obstruction neonatally, congenital heart disease, leukemia, and thyroid disease (Warkany, Passarge, & Smith, 1966). Parents may ask about the short stature and frequent respiratory infections associated with the disorder; these topics may be less psychologically threatening to them than the more serious issues.

Because heart disease is present in about 30% of DS infants, this usually comes up for discussion. The parents are informed that the major cause of mortality in DS is heart disease; most heart disease is found by the third month. With the advent of heart surgery and the control of numerous infectious dieases, life expectancy of DS individuals is increasing. Before the development of pediatric heart surgery, approximately one-half of DS children lived to 5 years of age. Once the child is 5, the chances are approximately .91 of reaching a normal life expectancy (Lilienfield, 1969).

Discussion of minor anomalies is often a focus of the parents' attention. They ask the counselor's opinion about these anomalies saying that they fail to see much difference between their child and other (normal) children. They seem to be hoping that the failure to find some particular anomaly will undo the diagnosis. Others will see the anomalies but will have located a friend or a relative with the same feature, also hoping to raise doubt as to the validity of the diagnosis. Not infrequently, a counselee might state that the baby seems perfectly normal. It is appropriate, at this point, to reassure them that for the first year of life the baby will behave almost like any other baby. This reassurance indicates to the parents that their perceptions are reliable, that the counselor is listening to them and is not trying to force something unbelievable on them. This latter point is particularly relevant when dealing with groups with whom medical personnel have traditionally had low credibility.

The interest and concern about the epicanthic folds, the brushfield, and the abnormal configuration of the helix of the ear are attempts on the part of the parents to organize their understanding of data they have into a meaningful picture. This is an important area for the counselor to understand and to interpret correctly in order to respond sensitively and effectively. If the concentration with the minor anomalies appears to be a means of avoiding the diagnosis, then an attempt to facilitate an integrated, intellectual conceptualization at this point would be inappropriate. The counselor needs to avoid confrontation with the counselees over this issue. Rather, the counselor should explore the meaning of the diagnosis and their interpretation of the facts with them.

Sometimes a counselee will want a detailed explanation of chromosome mechanics on the first visit. When I sense that this is their way of handling their anxiety (and when I feel that it is premature to explore the cause of their upset), I may provide a more detailed genetic explanation than usual. The *two* occasions on which I recall that counselees wanted detailed genetic explanations they seemed to use intellectualization as a means of coping and, in both cases, appeared to have difficulty accepting their child's diagnosis. Usually, I do not provide a detailed genetic explanation because most counselees appear uninterested in such facts and because facts that cause high anxiety are blocked out, especially until the diagnosis is confirmed by chromosomal studies.

Courses of treatment of the DS child also need to be discussed or are raised as issues for discussion by the counselees. The treatments for the major life threatening problems in DS are surgery for bowel obstruction in the neonatal period and heart surgery in infancy. Information needs to be provided as to the type of surgery available for these major malformations, the time it should and can be done, and an estimate of the success of the procedure. In addition, clear and detailed information about how to obtain consultation for surgery, when indicated, should be given.

When serious life threatening anomalies are diagnosed in a newborn with DS, many counselees question the advisability of surgery. In my experience, families with a baby who has gone home rarely raise this question, because the child has been incorporated into the family. However, when the problem is neonatal bowel obstruction and the baby has not yet been discharged from the hospital the potential for not choosing surgery exists and, indeed, is sometimes the parents' desired option. I believe that this is a legitimate issue to raise with parents. One way of approaching this subject is to tell the parents about how another family considered this option with the child dying before a decision could be made. By communicating this information to the parents, the counselor suggests that he or she is open to discussing the matter without suggesting a course of action. A counseling objective with families who choose not to have life prolonging intervention, is to help the counselees make a considered decision in which they articulate their guilt feelings. As an in-depth exploration of these feelings requires considerable counseling experience and skill, it is recommended that a person working full-time in psychological counseling participate in facilitating the decision and helping the counselees assess both the long-term and short-term consequences of their decision. Careful evaluation leading to a decision may lessen the emergence of later guilt.

Second Clinic Visit

The second clinic visit is geared to the confirmation of the diagnosis and the subsequent provision of genetic education. If it has not been obtained on the first visit, a psychosocial interview is carried out at this time. This is followed by a redefinition of their agendas in preparation for developing a counseling contract between the counselor and the counselees. When these are completed, then counselor and counselees begin to attend to the subjects on the agenda.

I begin by asking the counselees what they would like to accomplish during the counseling sessions. I make a written list of their concerns and then I tell them the things I think should be covered in the counseling. If there is a discrepancy, then it needs to be worked out before progressing. Our agendas usually coincide and so we have a basis for going on with the counseling. I then begin with the issues raised by the counselees. Frequently, this means postponing the explanation and discussion of the chromosomes to the end of the session. However, I am impressed that when this occurs, the counselees' motivation to hear and learn the genetics is enhanced.

The Counseling Process

The objectives of genetic counseling for parents with a child with DS depend on their actual level of knowledge about the diagnosis, the nature of the disorder, its prognosis, recurrence risk, prenatal diagnosis, available treatment, fertility control, and sources of help. For each assessment about the counselees' level of understanding, a judgment is made as to what the ideal level of their knowledge should be. The differential between these two levels defines the educational need. A decision is then made as to the tactical approaches to take to accomplish the immediate and overall educational objectives. The process is one of giving information, evaluating the counselee's knowledge, and observing their reactions to the information. Frequently, during the course of genetic education, the counselee becomes confused and attendant signs of anxiety may appear which halts the effective communication of information. An increase in anxiety connotes that the counselee understood the information and has been confronted with an awareness of its threatening implications. The counselor must then decide whether or not to discontinue giving facts and work toward lowering anxiety. The use of this process develops an effective rhythm of information giving and attending to emotional upset.

Information giving cannot always proceed to completion because of the normal anxiety arising from an immediate confrontation with bad news. When this happens, it is reasonable to answer questions and attempt to be supportive without compounding the stress with further facts unless there is some emergency in which the parents need to participate in a decision.

As the counseling progresses, the counselees are asked to repeat the various facts to determine whether and when they have learned them. The educational objectives are cognitive. They constitute the first evaluative sign indicative of progress towards psychological acceptance. According to the grief model of adaptation to change, the cognitive appreciation of the change is accompanied by anxiety (Falex, 1975; Antley, 1976; Macintyre, 1977). As acceptance progresses, hostility and depression may occur; these provide collateral data for evaluating the effects of the information at the emotional level. Emotional upset is ancillary information and is important in evaluating the application of genetic knowledge to decision making.

At the end of genetic education, the knowledge which the counselees attain raises issues, clarifies options in a probabilistic sense, and/or provides a more accurate basis for evaluating outcomes. The counselor, seeking an internally evaluated counselee decision will consider, conjointly with the counselees, the consequence of the alternative options for handling the situation. For a selected number of issues, the counselor needs to provide an opportunity for the counselee to rehearse the decision making. By the time this process is finished, the counselees should have had an opportunity to examine the outcome of their various options. Also, as the parents engage in their decision process a final and informative evaluation of the effectiveness of the counseling can be carried out by the counselor.

The concern with the educational task need not detract from attention to the emotional issues. By systematically dealing with the issues and simultaneously raising the counselees' awareness of their affective responses, it is more likely that they will become educated to their counseling needs. As this develops, contracting for further counseling may be indicated.

In spite of the planning of counseling approaches, a large part of the counselor's decisions as to how to proceed are made in dynamic response to the counselees and occurs in the midst of the process of the counseling session. Such decisions might be improved by formulating and planning beforehand and by postcounseling review.

Understanding the Counselee's Pain

In general, the outlook of a parent with a child with DS is that of a person who has suffered grievous losses or disappointments (Solnit & Stark, 1962) particularly centered on the anticipated health and intellectual function of his or her child. In addition, since people generally assume that they will procreate normal children, the fact that they have not may imply that their ability to have normal children is defective, leading to further feelings of loss or disappointment. The counselees' psychological reactions emanate from the meaning that the loss has for the individual. These meanings are generally bound up in the individual's concepts of self and in the constructs that the person holds as essential evidence for self worth as a person.

In our society, the belief in romantic love and marriage is often accompanied by the concept of an ideal, or at least, a normal family. The children in such families are expected to be a source of affection, pleasure, and pride. The birth of a child with DS is in opposition to these expectations. With the diagnosis of DS, one's sense of self and of family may be perceived as defective. No previous allowances other than of the idealized self and family have existed. Out of the disappointment which inevitably follows, a conflict emerges between the idealized and realized selves. The personal and family adjustments necessary to integrate and attempt to bring back into equilibrium the ideal self and the perceived self is the grief work.

The resolution of the conflict between the ideal and perceived selves is a painful process in which the parents oscillate between altering their identity to accomodate to the facts of having an affected child, and/or improving their estimate of the child's present and future functioning. Efforts to disregard the new information about the child might be thought of as attempts to maintain the previously held self-identity.

Sometimes, things are made more difficult by the fact that pregnancies are unwanted for part or all of the pregnancy. When this occurs, feelings of guilt may be mixed together with the feelings of disappointment, loss, and grief. The fact that the unwanted pregnancy bears no logical relation to the occurrence of DS is of little consequence. In our society, where individualism, self-responsibility, and the belief in cause and effect relationships are overriding themes, counselees often behave as if they had some culpability in having had a child with DS. The counselor needs to be sensitive to the counselee's pain; to its existence, its strength, and the counselee's vulnerability. These feelings are usually so intense that even under the best of circumstances they may go unarticulated after several hours of counseling.

Genetic Information

In providing genetic information, I begin with simple concepts and build to more complex ones in a stepwise fashion, always striving for the vocabulary which is at the counselee's educational level. I usually draw and write as I go, providing the counselee with a permanent record. Nondisjunction is explained as an accident of nature which occurs with great frequency in sexual reproduction. The frequency of recurrence is given as approximately 1/70 (Milunsky, 1973; Hamerton, 1976). Other relatives have the same risk as the population, about 1/1000.

When the child is found to have a translocation, the parents' chromosomes are also studied. In approximately three-fourths of the cases the chromosomes are normal. The parents are reassured that the translocation was a new mutational event with a recurrence risk of less than 2%. When, however, the counselees are carriers of a translocation, they are shown their karyotype as well as that of the child at the time of counseling. If the mother is the carrier they are given a recurrence risk of approximately 10%; if the father, then the risk is approximately 5% (Kikuchi, Oisni, Tonomura, 1969). In addition, the family is told of the inherited nature of the translocation so that chromosome studies can be done in other relatives who might be carriers.

Options for Dealing with the Recurrence Risk

The options open to counselees dealing with their risk of recurrence depend on the couples' fertility plans. A list of possible counselee decisions and corresponding behaviors is presented to the counselees for their review (Table 7.1). This decision chart has a number of advantages. Because it is printed and impersonal, the counselee is unlikely to interpret the discussion of these issues as the counselor suggesting a course of action. In addition, it clarifies the options and leads to a systematic, thorough review of the alternatives. For counselees who are fertile, a decision about fertility control is inescapable. The decision chart leads logically to evaluating the consequence of a decision and of fertility control behavior.

Information on various types of birth control is available from family planning centers. It needs to be ascertained whether or not the counselees have knowledge about how to get information to control their own fertility. For counselees who consider a future pregnancy, there is the additional option of prenatal diagnosis. Even if they oppose abortion, it is usually a good idea to provide the counselees with the facts on amniocentesis.

The primary purpose of having prenatal diagnosis is to provide the couple with the reassurance that they are carrying a chromosomally normal fetus. However, if it turns out that they are not, they still have an opportunity to make a decision about whether to continue the pregnancy. There are advantages to knowing ahead of time that an affected infant will be born and that the danger of fetal loss or stillborn exists. Parents and physicians have an opportunity to organize their resources and to experience less shock after the child's birth and to anticipate grief. Experience with prenatal diagnosis has shown that both people who say they will terminate and those who say they will not terminate have changed their minds after obtaining antenatal chromosome reports on their fetus (Hamerton, 1976). Thus, it is advisable to provide information on prenatal diagnosis to all counselees, regardless of who plans to utilize it.

Experience has shown that reviewing the potential outcome of prenatal

Table 7.1
Counselee Decisions For Fertility Planning [a]

	Start	Yes	No
1.	Do you plan to have a child?	Proceed	Go to 8
2.	Do you plan to refrain from birth control at this time?	Proceed	Go to 10
3.	Do you want a child now?	Proceed	Go to 12
4.	PROCEED WITH EDUCATION ABOUT PRENATAL DIAGNOSIS		
5.	PROCEED WITH FERTILITY		
6.	Do you wish to utilize prenatal diagnosis?	Proceed	Go to 14
7.	PROCEED WITH PRENATAL DIAGNOSIS PROCEDURE STOP: Decision making complete		
8.	Do you wish to have sterilization?	Proceed	Go to 2
9.	PROCEED WITH STERILIZATION PROCEDURE STOP: Decision making complete		
10.	PROCEED WITH EDUCATION ABOUT BIRTH CONTROL		
11.	Have you changed your decision to use birth control?	Go to 1	STOP: Decision making complete
12.	DANGEROUS SITUATION—DISCUSS WITH COUNSELOR THEN PROCEED	STOP: Decision making complete	Go to 1
13.	Are undependable means of birth control (abstinence, abortion, etc.) acceptable options for you?		
14.	Do you accept the risk?	STOP: Decision making complete	Go to 12

[a] To use the decision chart, start at the top and proceed through each number unless your answer (yes or no) indicates otherwise or until decision making is complete.

diagnosis may be a good way of checking the counselee's understanding of the recurrence risk. I set up the alternative outcomes of the studies and ask them to provide the probabilities. Poor understanding and misunderstanding, if they exist, usually emerge during the session on a straightforward need-to-know basis which allows further genetic education without raising undue defensiveness.

Developmental Issues

A major problem which needs to be discussed is the issue of mental retardation. Parents need to have a general description of intellectual function in DS so as to have a basis for reasonable future expectations. Parents are informed that the level of attainment of any individual is uncertain but that on the average the person with DS is in the range of moderate retardation.

The counselor needs to be specific in describing the state of moderate retardation, relating it, whenever possible, to tasks about which the parents have first hand information. In discussing the development of an infant with DS, I usually proceed through the various developmental milestones, giving the parents the range with which they might expect to deal.

To ascertain the specific level of their child's performance, intelligence testing alone is discouraged. Rather, continuous progress evaluation and goal setting is recommended. The child should be evaluated on his or her specific level of gross motor and fine motor control, emotional maturity, and language skills. On the basis of attainment and progress over the previous interval of time, professionals and parents might set goals which have a 70–80% chance of attainment during the forthcoming interval. Continuous progress evaluations provide parents with realistic perspectives, and it has a built-in success factor which might promote the child's motivation. Lastly, it removes the inexorable sense of fate that is so often extrapolated from IQ scores.

In the area of preschool education, I generally answer questions in general terms. The counselor needs to be aware of the educational opportunities available in the counselee's community. For children with DS there are early intervention programs in many communities that send personnel to the home and begin working with the parents as early as 6 months after delivery. I often refer children and their families to community agencies which can provide them with the ongoing help they need.

I generally point out the advantages that early educational programs provide. These include an increased development of social skills and better behavior control as DS children reach school age and beyond. I underscore the point that better social skills tend to lead to greater public acceptance of the person with DS and consequently, a higher effective intelligence. Associations for retarded citizens provide education for parents so that in our community the virtually undisciplined child with DS is a rarity. In addition to preschool programs, vocational training is also available through these agencies.

The opportunity for parent education by observing individuals with DS of all ages is also significant educational potential. Many parents with a new baby with DS have no information or a limited experience with the disorder. Visiting the preschool and sheltered workshops may provide parents with a clearer description of future expectations than is possible from words alone. Most parents are not ready for this type of confrontation for several months or more after the birth of the child, but when they are, it is a valuable extension of the educational process started in genetic counseling.

With respect to the issue of sexuality in the DS individual, I deal with this only if it is raised by the counselees. I do so because of the limited time available and the remoteness of the concern from their present situation.

Evaluating the Outcome

As the parents engage in their decision process, a final and informative evaluation of the effectiveness of the counseling can be carried out by the counselor. Successful genetic counseling shows evidence (a) that the negative feelings of the counselee have diminished as the grief process progresses towards resolution; (b) that the counselee approaches decision making by defining options and evaluating them from multiple perspectives; (c) that the counselee's behavior is in keeping with the decisions and he is acting responsibly.

Good Case Management

The thesis of good case management is to bring together the relevant helpful options for the child and the family. To accomplish this goal, I write out the information covered in the counseling session and, in addition, send a letter covering this material to the family after the counseling session. Finally, if they accept referral to another agency, a form letter to the agency is typed on their behalf. They can sign the letter if they wish and the genetics assistant sends it on to the agency. This increases the success rate in referral and reduces the waiting time for further help.

Another aim of good case management is to garner the facilities from the total health care system that might be needed for the family. Someone often needs to coordinate these activities. If it is found that no one is doing this and the family is on a random course, then part of the management is at least temporarily coordinating the care from multiple sources.

Obviously, all counselees do not continue counseling or, for that matter, even keep the first appointment. This is usually a sign of distress and destructive repression and denial. When this occurs, an attempt is made to reschedule the appointment and the referring physician is called. The relationship with the parents is often such that the physician can facilitate the referral. Conversely, if the physician is not kept abreast of developments, he or she can have an extraordinary influence in reinforcing the denial. At the least, the referring physician needs to be kept informed. It is essential to good case management that both the referring physician and the counselor have compatible facts. If rescheduling the parents is unsuccessful, then an attempt is made to stay in telephone contact. Because of grief dynamics, some counselees will not complete counseling. It is important to understand their feelings and not take the rejection of services in a personal way. The repeated expression of concern and openness to potential counselees is the genetic counselor's access to forming a counseling relationship. This relationship becomes the counselees' access to treatment.

Role of the Counselor

The counselor's presence in genetic counseling humanizes it and differentiates it from nonhuman or inanimate types of educational processes. It is this human component which helps the counselees deal with their own personal situation, the realities of having a child with DS, the susceptibility of the child and family for further morbidity, and the benefits and costs of exercising various options. In general, the more the counselees believe that the counselor understands their predicament, strengths, liabilities, and goals and accepts their feelings, the greater will be their trust in the counselor. The counselees will not only share more about themselves, they will also be more likely to be willing to confront situations in which an active decision will lead to a sense of control over their lives.

Two factors help the counselor enter into a trusting therapeutic relationship with the counselees: knowledge and counseling skills. The reason the counselee seeks a relationship with the counselor is because the counselor has access to a restricted body of knowledge, namely, the medical and genetic information. Almost invariably, counselees come to the genetic counseling clinic with a wider range of questions than that concerning the genetic aspects of DS. The ability of the counselor to respond knowledgeably and flexibly to the counselee's questions provides a basis which allows their relationship to develop. The counselor attempts to begin where the counselee is ready to work, to build rapport at this level and ultimately to cover the majority of important content issues during the counseling.

The counselor also needs to have and to develop a knowledge of the counselee as a person. Knowing and referring to the counselee by name may be a start. Beyond this, it is often helpful to find out details about the parents' closest relatives and support group. It may be easier to talk about matters about which the counselee is familiar as part of the process of getting acquainted. Taking time to learn this casual information about the counselee cannot be underrated. The counselor's knowledge of the counselees' social, educational, and financial setting, and of their life and work enable the counselor to relate to them better.

Among the counseling skills which promote the human relationship between the counselee and the genetic counselor are:

1. The counselor's unreserved acceptance of the counselee
2. his or her sensitivity and constructive honesty
3. his or her initiative in staying "in relationship" with the counselees
4. the ability to make meaningful interventions into destructive patterns of counselee behavior.

Since these skills are discussed elsewhere in this volume, I will comment briefly on the counselor's capacity for acceptance and sensitivity to what the counselees are trying to communicate.

Counselor Characteristics

The acceptance of another is a characteristic which facilitates human relationships; it is crucial in genetic counseling. The type of acceptance I have in mind is an unconditional regard for the counselees as people and for their feelings. It includes the acceptance of the counselees' feelings and concerns even when by objective standards the concern or feeling appears to be in excess of the actual danger. Also, the counselor strives to accept the counselees' negative feelings about themselves, their child and even about the counselor. It is not a matter of agreeing or disagreeing but rather an acceptance of the counselees' right to have their feelings and to make their own decisions. The counselor may actually disagree with the decision and may, if an adequate relationship exists, tell the counselees that he or she disagrees. However, the counselor should always attempt to understand the reasoning of the counselees and empathize with their feelings on the subject. To be empathic means that the counselor must have sensitive listening skills.

There are many reasons why the genetic counselor needs to develop listening skills. Such skills provide the means to maintain the relationship with the counselees. The counselor's sensitivity helps the counselor be more effective in providing genetic education, in facilitating the counselees' decision-making process and in assessing the counselees' level of anxiety. If their anxiety is too high, the counselor will need to work towards its reduction. If too low, the counselor may wish to let the counselees' anxiety build so that there is more motivation for the counselee to take charge of the problems arising out of the birth of a child with DS.

In general, when new information is given or confrontation is offered, the counselees' anxiety will rise. Sometimes the counselees may wish to move on to additional information as a means of avoiding the anxiety produced by the original material. For this reason, the counselor may need to stop from time to time and ask the counselees to summarize what has been covered. When anxiety is high the chances are that the counselees will have the facts confused, a phenomenon previously noted by Money (1975). In addition to repeating the content information, the counselees should be asked to evaluate the facts for their child and themselves. This engages the counselees in assigning meaning to the information and articulating their feelings about it. To the extent that the counselees can come to an understanding of what they are feeling and relate it to behavior that they can modify if they so choose, the more the counselees will feel that they are in control of their lives. Failure of the counselees to achieve this understanding tends to leave the counselees in a poor psychological state for decision making.

Many genetic counselors are untrained in psychological counseling. At the same time they are placed into situations where they need the ability to listen to the counselees and to understand them on an emotional level. There are a number of ways counselors might improve their listening and counseling skills. For example, tape recordings of genetic counseling sessions is an inexpensive way of obtaining a record of what occurred in the session and may be used to obtain individual or group supervision from competent professionals. At a minimum, the counselors might listen to their own tapes and attempt to evaluate their performance with such scales as those developed by Carkhuff (1969).

Appendix

PSYCHOSOCIAL WORKUP

The psychosocial workup includes an evaluation of the degree to which the counselees are able to affirm themselves. Also it provides an estimate of the strength of the relationship with their partner. Finally, an evaluation is made of how the parents are progressing in their coping with the stress arising from the fact that their child has DS. This information guides the way in which the counselor approaches the counseling task. Prior to meeting with the counselees, the staff meets to discuss the psychosocial evaluation. A counseling strategy is agreed upon which takes into account the counselees' history of self affirmation, sources of support out of the parents relationship and where the counselees are in their process of grieving.

In the workup, the counselees are interviewed separately by a person with skills in psychological counseling. An evaluation of self esteem is made and the family dynamics and the patterns of interaction with others, of handling conflict, and of dealing with emotions are determined. Open-ended questions are asked to elicit specific information and also to shed light on the person's general sources of affirmation, the degree of satisfaction within the relationship, and how anger is handled. For example, inquiring about the things the counselees enjoy and from which they receive satisfaction often reveals something about the sources of the counselees' affirmation. The self-affirming counselees are internally supporting and resistant to the opinion of others in evaluating themselves. Some counselees evaluate themselves according to social norms, as for example, the person who obtains affirmation from his or her professional identity. Others seek the affirmation of their family and comport themselves so as to receive reinforcement from their spouse, parents, or other parent-like figures. The more internal and self-affirming a person is, the more resistant he or she is to feelings of self guilt, shame, and low self-concept. The random and self destructive behavior parents sometimes manifest after having a child with DS can often be related to ways in which their usual sources of affirmation are perceived to have been interrupted.

In addition to assessing the individual's strength and resilience, the potential for support in the relationship with the spouse is evaluated. To accomplish this, the degree of satisfaction within the marriage is explored. When the counselees report satisfaction in their relationship, additional exploration is needed because such responses may be perceived as socially desirable. When the response is one of low satisfaction, the counselor probably has obtained valid information; the candor of this answer suggests that the counselees will be open to talking about these and other problems in greater detail. If the male counselee reports being in a marriage with little satisfaction, then he might consider himself as being "trapped" in the relationship if the child has DS. The counselor should look for anger, desperation, bewilderment, and behaviors that lead to greater levels of uncertainty, frustration, and sadness for the counselee. The counselor should also be alerted that in addition to genetic counseling, family or marriage counseling needs to be offered and encouraged as a part of the extended counseling treatment design.

If the mother reports low satisfaction in the marriage, further information is needed to estimate her probable response to the diagnosis. If she enjoys taking care of children and sees her role as the "good mother," then having a child with DS may present little threat. She may even see it as enhancing her enjoyment of mothering and perhaps adding stability to an otherwise precarious marital relationship. Conversely, if this is her first child or if she sees her role as including significant activities other than mothering, then the woman's reaction will probably be analogous to that of the man.

When the counselee reports satisfaction from the partnership, it may mean either (a) that the relationship is one in which there is growing intimacy, respect, and individuality, (b) that it reflects a satisfaction derived from the gratification of dependency needs, or (c) it is a socially desirable response. To clarify these possibilities, the counselor may seek to determine how decisions are made by the couple. Again, the counselor needs to listen carefully because sometimes the woman will report that the husband makes the decision when actually she does and vice versa. In this instance, obtaining specific information about how some recent decisions were made and the relative amount of individual input into these decisions might clarify their behavior patterns.

Another important task is to evaluate how anger is handled in the relationship. This can be accomplished by asking if anger between the partners is dangerous. If the answer is no and/or the counselee can articulate how anger and frustration are put to constructive use in the relationship, this may be taken as evidence for strength in the relationship (Smith & Antley, 1978).

Since, in addition to the emotional burden, caring for a child with DS is generally difficult and time-consuming, the counselor might expect marital problems to develop in "satisfactory" relationships in which there is a dependent member. The obligatory dependency of the child with DS is likely to detract from the dependent counselee's satisfaction. Also, having a child with DS leads to a certain amount of frustration. If the expression of anger between the mates is taboo, either the relationship will break down under the stress or a period of personal growth and maturity may result. The counselor may be instrumental in helping couples in either situation.

The results of the psychosocial evaluations tend to fall into relatively consistent patterns. For example, individuals who are internally oriented tend to be found in relationships which are also resistant to external stress and to breakdowns in communications. Conversely, persons who seek their affirmation from parents and parent-like figures tend to be dependent. Out of their need to have others think well of them, they will tend to dampen and withhold expression of their anger. The information collected during the precounseling interview helps to identify those individuals who are most likely to have difficulty with the genetic counseling and with having to adapt to a child with DS.

The psychosocial workup also provides an opportunity to assess how well the person and the family are coping with the emotional aspect of the genetic diagnosis and an estimate as to how receptive a counselee might be to the information of genetic counseling. Two factors are taken into account:

1. The degree to which previously supplied information has been assimilated
2. How he or she is managing the stress of the diagnosis.

If the counselees are actively denying as a way of dealing with the diagnosis, then the counselor may want to go more slowly with information-giving and attempt to extend the counseling over a number of sessions. Counseling can move more quickly when the counselees use anxiety to motivate their behavior and when they have control over the behavior.

Acknowledgments

I am indebted to Keith Kinney, Th.M., who has carefully and constructively criticized the development of this counseling program and suggested many helpful avenues of approach over the two years of its development. Kenneth E. Reed, Ph.D., and George Siskind, Ph.D., have given intensive assistance in conceptualizing and refining the model. Mary Ann Antley, Alex Braitman, Peg Goldberg and Seymour Kessler, Ph.D., have given able assistance in reviewing drafts.

References

Antley, R. M. Variables in the outcome of genetic counselng. *Social Biology*, 1976, 23, 108–115.
Antley, R. M. Factors influencing mother's responses to genetic counseling for Down's syndrome. In *Genetic counseling*, Felix de la Cruz & Herbert A. Lubs, (Eds.), New York: Raven Press, 1977.
Carkuff, R. *Helping and human relations*, (Vol. 1 & 2). New York: Holt, Rinehart, and Winston, 1969.
Falek, A. J. Applications of the coping process to genetic counseling. Presented at the Genetics Counseling Meeting, Colorado Springs, Colorado, February 26–27, 1975.

Hamerton, J. L. Perspectives on prenatal diagnosis from U.S.A. and Canada amniocentesis registries. *Excerpta Medica ICS*, 1976, 397, 9.

Horrobin, J. M., & Rynders, J. E. *To give an edge*. Minneapolis, Minnesota: The Colwell Press, 1975.

Kikuchi, Y., Oisni, H., Tonomura, A., Yamada, K., Tanaka, Y., Kurita, T., & Matsunaga, E. Translocation Down's syndrome in Japan: Its frequency, mutation rate of translocation and parental age. *Japanese Journal of Human Genetics*, 1969, *14*(2), 93–106.

Lilienfield, A. Epidemiology of mongolism. Baltimore: The Johns Hopkins Press, 1969.

Macintyre, M. N. Need for supportive therapy for members of a family with a defective child. In *Genetic counseling*, Felix de la Cruz & Herbert A. Lubs, (Eds.), New York: Raven Press, 1977.

Milunsky, A. *The prenatal diagnosis of hereditary disorders*. Springfield, Illinois: Thomas Publishers, 1973.

Money, J. Counseling in genetics and applied behavior genetics. In *Developmental human behavior genetics*, K. W. Schaie, V. E. Anderson, G. E. McLearns, & J. Money, (Eds.), Lexington, Massachusetts: Lexington Books, 1975.

Roboz, P. & Pitt, D. Studies on 782 cases of mental deficiency, Part III. *The Australian Paediatric Journal*, 1969, *5*, 38–53.

Smith, R. W., & Antley, R. M. Anger: A significant obstacle to informed decision making in genetic counseling, birth defects: Original Articles Series, 1978. In press.

Solnit, A. J. & Stark, M. H. Mourning and the birth of a defective child. *The Psychoanalytic Study of the Child Journal*, 1962, *16*, 523–537.

Warkany, J., Passarge, E. & Smith, L. B. Congenital malformations in autosomal trisomy syndromes. *American Journal of Diseases of Children*, 1966, *112*, 502–517.

Psychological Issues in Genetic Counseling of Phenylketonuria

8

Sylvia Schild

Phenylketonuria (PKU) is the classic model for the study of inborn errors of metabolism. The opportunity for primary prevention of mental retardation through neonatal screening and dietary treatment was hailed as a significant breakthrough at a time when little was known about causes and treatment of mental retardation. Initially, major focus was placed on early identification, diagnosis, and medical management of the PKU child. Basic research efforts were directed toward a search for new knowledge about the biochemical nature of the metabolic error in PKU. Clinical research and interest has centered primarily on the efficacy of dietary treatment and on the factors related to intelligence. With an ever enlarging pool of treated cases, some interest has been shown in the personality and behavior of the PKU child. Although psychological research has been minimal, some evidence suggests that PKU individuals have intellectual and perceptual defects reducing their coping strategies for dealing with life tasks and stress. Even less study has been undertaken of the family of the PKU child and the impact of the disorder on the family (Schild, 1968). In general, the overriding concerns of parents and professionals alike center on the medical care of the PKU child and the development of the child's mental status. These concerns are inextricably intertwined with the daily demands and exigencies of the dietary treatment. Only superficial recognition has been given to the stresses engendered by the hereditary nature of PKU for the family. Partly, this was so because of a lack of interest in the dynamics of genetic counseling. It is only recently that specific attention is being directed toward an

135

GENETIC COUNSELING
Psychological Dimensions

enlightened understanding of how genetic information is imparted and comprehended and toward an appreciation of its effects on the lives of genetically affected indivduals and their families.

This chapter is organized in two major sections. The first section presents facts about phenylketonuria (PKU) germaine to the issues and problems dealt with in genetic counseling. The second section discusses the consequences of PKU for the affected individual and the family. This material is presented within a framework which views genetic disorders from a crisis perspective; implications for facilitating a positive adaptation to the problem of PKU will be noted.

The Genetics of PKU

PKU occurs in approximately 1 out of every 10,000 to 15,000 births. It affects primarily Caucasians, with the incidence being highest in Northern Europe and the United States, and is very rare in African, Jewish, and Finnish populations. The defect is transmitted by an autosomal recessive gene; therefore, the affected individual receives an abnormal gene from each of his parents. Unaffected parents are heterozygous carriers and with each pregnancy there is a one in four chance that the child will be affected.

It is possible to identify carriers as a group by means of phenylalanine tolerance tests; however, it is not possible to determine zygosity accurately in individual cases. This inability to determine carrier status makes it impossible to counsel with specificity regarding the recurrence risks for unaffected siblings of a PKU individual. The best one can do, at present, is emphasize the rare incidence of the disorder and stress the very slim probabilistic risks of carriers mating. It is estimated that one in 50 in the Caucasian population is a carrier of the recessive gene for PKU; in Blacks, the incidence is about one in 250. The risk for a PKU child in carrier X carrier marriages is roughly 1 in 2500 among Caucasians.

Dietary Treatment

The treatment for the PKU child is a low phenylalanine diet. At the same time, the diet must contain an adequate amount of phenylalanine essential for normal growth and development. Since phenylalanine is found in all protein-rich foods, the dietary treatment is very restrictive— fish, meats, poultry, eggs, milk, bread products are all excluded; hence, the need for a special preparation to provide essential nutrients. Lofenalac®

is the major product used to fill the protein needs of the growing child. Other products such as Albumaid, Aminagran, and Cymogran are also available but not extensively used in the United States.

The dietary prescriptions are based on the child's age and tolerance for phenylalanine. In addition to the synthetic formula, the diet includes foods from a free list of nonprotein calories. Serving lists, comparable to diabetic exchange lists, have been prepared for use of families and professionals working with PKU families (Acosta, Schaeffler, Wenz, & Koch, 1972).

Successful dietary treatment depends on the parents' management of the child and on their understanding of the disease and the diet requirements. It also depends on the child's understanding of the diet restrictions and on the self-discipline of the child. Problems in dietary control are related to either too little or too much intake of phenylalanine. The problems stem from physiologic factors such as acute illnesses, weight loss, failure to gain, and from environmental causes such as "snitching" by the PKU child, feeding patterns of parents and other caretakers, and errors in instruction of the diet prescription. Factors in the family situation influencing the dietary control are often of crucial importance and require exploration after all medical considerations have been examined.

Doubt still exists as to when dietary therapy should be terminated. The current trend leans towards discontinuance at about 6–8 years of age. The rationale is that this is the period when myelination and brain mass have reached the level present at maturity. Greater reservations prevail about diet discontinuance for girls because of the data on mentally retarded offspring of PKU mothers.

Newborn Screening Programs

It is not possible to detect PKU prenatally by amniocentesis; the next best thing is to identify the patient as early as possible such as at birth. The development of the Guthrie inhibition Assay for phenylalanine made mass neonatal screening programs possible. Legislation establishing mandatory testing of the newborn has been passed in 44 of the United States (President's Committee on Mental Retardation, 1976) and newborn screening programs exist world-wide. Although legal and ethical issues have been raised about mandatory testing, at this point in time, the benefits derived from mandatory screening seem to hold sway. For example, since newborn screening began in California in 1966, not one child with a diagnosis of PKU has been admitted to an institution for the mentally retarded (R. Koch, personal communication).

The test for PKU is usually done on the day of discharge from the newborn nursery. When a presumptive positive test for PKU is made, the child is hospitalized for diagnostic evaluation and pedigree information is obtained. Generally, serum phenylalanine levels are obtained on parents, siblings, and other available relatives. Treatment is implemented if the diagnosis of PKU is confirmed. In some centers, a challenge test is carried out at a subsequent time for reconfirmation of the diagnosis. Genetic counseling is initiated, generally, when a firm diagnosis has been made.

A frequent question asked of the genetic counselor relates to the reproductive risks for the affected individual. In the past, this issue was of negligible importance as most untreated PKU cases became severely retarded and were institutionalized. However, as successful treatment proceeds, PKU individuals are increasingly marrying and attempting to raise children of their own. All of the children of a PKU individual will be obligate carriers, if the mating is with a noncarrier. The mating between an affected person and a heterozygote would produce one half affecteds and one half carriers. Should two PKU homozygotes mate, all their offspring would be affected. If matings are random, the chances of this happening would be very small. However, this risk may increase as the pool of treated PKU individuals grows and as families have increased contacts with each other through clinics and parent groups.

Maternal PKU

In addition to their genetic risks, several studies (Mabry, 1963; Mac-Cready & Levy, 1971) show that PKU mothers have an increased rate of abortion and an elevated risk for producing non-PKU offspring with mental retardation and multiple congenital anomalies, including microcephaly, growth retardation, congenital heart disease, and hemivertebra.

Theoretically, if PKU mothers remain on the low phenylalanine diet throughout their pregnancies and maintain a normal range of serum phenylalanine levels, they should be able to produce normal offspring. Two successful cases have been reported (Arthur & Hulme, 1970; Mac-Cready & Levy, 1971); however, followup assessment is needed to determine whether these children will develop normally. Most experience with Maternal PKU has had ominous overtones. The mothers were unable to maintain the diet, had consistently elevated serum phenylalanine levels, and produced severely defective children. Counseling generally has been slanted toward the recommendation of solutions other than natural childbearing; that is, sterilization, therapeutic abortion if conception has already occurred, and adoption if children are wanted. On the basis of current knowledge, the possibility of Maternal PKU as the etiology of undiagnosed mental retardation in multiple members of a family should not be overlooked.

Psychological Aspects

Mental development in most PKU children appears to be inversely related to the age at which the dietary treatment is begun (Shear, Willman & Nyhan, 1974). Children who are diagnosed later than the newborn period tend to show some intellectual impairment and need to be placed into special education classes. The most common learning problem involves tasks requiring visual-perceptual abilities. While children who have hyperphenylalaninemia show normal levels of intelligence, many of these also show mild to moderate degrees of visual-perceptual difficulties. One study of treated PKU children which used normal siblings as matched-pair controls suggests that when treatment begins early and is rigorously monitored, there is a small but statistically significant intellectual impairment associated with PKU (Dobson, Kushida, Williamson, & Friedman, unpublished).

Children with PKU are frequently reported to show behavioral abnormalities, communication defects, and extreme hyperactivity. PKU children tend to show greater variability in interactional behavior than groups of normal children, mentally retarded children, and children who are psychotic (Steisel, Friedman, Wood, & Steisel, 1967). Recent studies suggest that experiential factors may be implicated in the occurrence of reported behavioral abnormalities (Friedman, Wood & Steisel, 1967; Friedman, Sibinga, Steisel, & Sinnamon, 1968; Koch, Blaskovics, Wenz, Fishler, & Schaeffler, 1974). Mothers of PKU children tend to be overprotective and to inhibit normal exploratory activity of their children. This dynamic has been noted in both food-related and nonfood-related situations and may account for some of the learning deficits observed in treated PKU children and for the deficits reported in verbal expression (Steisel, Katz & Harris, 1974).

There is considerable clinical evidence that the strict dietary treatment strongly affects the mother–child relationship and that the PKU child is likely to have many behavior problems which center around food. Behavior modification techniques have been used with some success to help parents cope with the behavioral difficulties of the PKU child.

The Phenylketonuric Family

A FRAMEWORK FOR VIEWING
THE GENETIC PROBLEM

To understand the psychological and social issues associated with PKU, a broadened perspective of what it means to have a serious genetic problem of any kind may be helpful. The characteristic aspects of a genetic problem influence, impinge on, and identify the nature of potential stresses and expectable responses experienced by affected members and their families. The dynamics of the psychological issues in the genetic counseling in PKU are no less impacted by these generic attributes than in other genetic disorders.

One obvious generic characteristic is the *permanency* of the genetic diagnosis. Once made, the genetic diagnosis *ipso facto* defines an irreversible condition, a problem that won't go away! The diagnosis of PKU is a point of no return—the family becomes once and forever distinguishable as a "PKU Family." The permanent nature of the genetic diagnosis has important psychological and situational implications for the family. For example, it means the taking on or integration of a new identity—as parent-of-a-PKU-child, as carrier-of-the-PKU-gene, as a person-with-PKU. The diagnosis may also signal the presence of a chronic disability. The lifelong nature of PKU may have a serious impact on the structure, development, and interactional processes of family life. The chronic nature of PKU may express itself as a threat at varying points in the life history of individuals and their families, for instance, in relation to significant events such as marriage. Thus, decision making about crucial life tasks and aspirations may be affected by the genetic concerns. In the PKU child's early life, the focus is on dietary treatment, the management of medical problems, and on intellectual development. In adolescence and young adulthood, attention shifts to marriage concerns and childbearing risks (especially with PKU girls). The long-term effects of dietary treatment are still an unknown, so prediction of psychosocial tasks and issues in advance maturity is not currently feasible.

The genetic disorder is characteristically a *family problem*; whenever heredity is implicated, family members automatically are identified as being at high risk. The diagnosis in one member may lead to the identification of others in the family who are homozygous for PKU. The genetic risks for other family members are identified. Additionally, the family is inevitably involved in the care and management of the PKU patient. In PKU, the efficacy of the dietary treatment is largely entrusted to the parents.

Another common feature of a genetic disorder is its inherent *complexity*.

This characteristic is noteworthy in PKU which has a highly complicated biochemical basis and whose differential diagnosis relates to complex metabolic processes. Because of its nature, communicating a clear understanding of the disease to individuals at risk is filled with difficulties. Most lay persons have limited scientific knowledge and comprehension of normal probability theory. Most professionals make the assumption that a clear understanding of PKU is essential to rational decision making around recurrence risks. The success in the management of the patient and the adequacy of the family's adjustment are also assumed to be directly related to how well the family comprehends the PKU information. In general, empiric studies (Wood, Friedman, & Steisel, 1967; Schild, 1968; Sibinga & Friedman, 1971; Leonard, Chase, & Childs, 1972) reveal that most parents of PKU children have marked tendencies to distort medical information or have difficulty clearly conceptualizing their child's illness despite careful and long-term instruction. Even when empirical measurements showed that parents were well informed, the interviews revealed gross distortions of the pertinent facts (Schild, 1968). For example, a common description given of PKU was: "It causes poison in the blood which is like an acid and eats away at (or burns holes in) the brain [p. 75]."

Most genetic counseling and information on PKU is provided at the time of diagnosis. This is a time when pertinent data is apt to be filtered through a screen of intense emotional responses generated by the diagnosis. It is not too surprising that the information is not clearly taken in and often distorted.

The uncertainties or ambiguities of establishing a differential diagnosis may interfere with effective genetic counseling. The span of time needed to make a differential diagnosis may compound the anxieties, fears, frustrations, and uncertainties of the family members; all of which complicates rationality of functioning and of thinking processes.

Another generic aspect of a genetic problem relates to the *labeling* that occurs. Granted, the necessity to label is of importance in detection, treatment, and prevention activities. Nevertheless, it also acts to identify a difference, a *deviance*, in the individual and the family. The impact of labeling on the person's self-image, in terms of self-adequacy, and self-esteem, can be momentous. Labeling engenders a sense of shame, partly in response to the social stigma which may be attached to the label. Stigmatization, in turn, may lead to social ostracism, which may engender a sense of isolation and alienation. An illustration of the dynamic impact of the labeling process is reflected in the statement of a mother of a PKU child who said: "I felt as if the diagnosis had been branded on my forehead . . . I think of it in every waking minute [Schild, 1968]."

Finally, and possibly the most significant characteristic of the genetic problem, the genetic diagnosis constitutes a *threat,* or *hazardous event* and may be perceived as a crisis precipitant. The diagnosis is a turning point upsetting the balance of family life and initiating a host of new problems—emotional and situational—that require resolution and call for coping strategies applicable to the new situation. The *meaning* attached to the hazardous event, to the PKU diagnosis for example, will in large part shape how the family will adapt to the crisis situation precipitated by the diagnosis.

There are many potential threats inherent in a genetic diagnosis. In some disorders the outcome can be fatal illness (in PKU, if untreated, infant death is a real possibility) or a shortened life span. The diagnosis may foretell chronic illness and disability (i.e., in PKU, mental retardation, seizures, learning disabilities). As a crisis precipitant, the genetic diagnosis may acutely assault established values held by the family. Many parents raise questions about their moral right to reproduce and possibly increase the pool of heterozygotes or risk having another PKU child. It is not uncommon to have parents question the ethics of prescribing a dietary treatment when the long range effects are unclear—is one problem being traded for another? Religious beliefs are vulnerable for challenge in some families, particularly in relation to family planning considerations.

The genetic diagnosis poses a real threat to the marital relationship of the parents, adding vulnerability to the sexual relationship and stressing family interactions. "It's your family who has the bad blood!" "The marriage was indeed or perhaps a mistake?" "Who wanted the child anyway?" These are common questions (overtly or covertly expressed) which reflect threats to marital stability as parents struggle with the intense emotional reactions to the diagnosis. Many parents report aroused fearfulness of engaging in sexual relations following the diagnosis. The feelings of personal failure of having produced a PKU child often permeate all aspects of the sexual relationship; avoidance and strained relations are common consequences. The fear of pregnancy thwarts and inhibits natural sexual responsiveness and intimacy. Marital and sexual conflicts generated by the PKU diagnosis tend to dissipate once the couple reach agreement about the genetic risks and arrive at a mutual decision with respect to future childbearing (Schild, 1968).

The implicit ego threats have already been mentioned. The self-blame and diminished self-esteem are apparent in this typical statement of a father of three PKU children: "I keep thinking of what I've done to my children. It doesn't make me feel good about myself." Implicitly evident is the parents' knowledge that what they have produced is an extension of themselves. This can have a devastating effect on the ego.

A threat emanating from genetic diagnosis relates to the loss that is implied or experienced, be it death, shortened life span, the anticipated fantasized child, identity, or preferred life style. The degree of loss experienced is contingent on the personalities of the involved individuals, the meanings given to the perceived losses, and the extent to which the families are in crisis.

In addition to the psychological threats inherent to the genetic diagnosis, many crises may occur as a result of external stresses. Burdensome reality factors, as well as the perceived burden of care may precipitate personal or family crises. The responsibility for managing the child's diet can be inordinately oppressive for some parents. Also, the pressures exerted by significant others and the attitudes and reactions of acquaintances, friends, and neighbors may be perceived or interpreted in ways which may trigger a family crisis. Financial demands, medical directives, agency requirements, etc., may all be critical stresses for families with genetic disorders.

When the genetic diagnosis is viewed as a hazardous event, a crisis model may be used to understand the behavior of families and to provide a framework for helping interventions and counseling. The awareness that PKU families will have both acute and chronic maturational and situational crises, complicated by the presence of the genetic defect makes it imperative to ascertain how families perceive the genetic event and, in general, how they respond and adapt to it. Exploratory evidence (Schild, 1968, unpublished) suggests that some parents of PKU children may have unstable personalities and function erratically, thus complicating the medical management of their children. One conjecture is that the parental instability exists by virtue of their being heterozygous for PKU. Another speculation is that the psychological impact of the diagnosis evokes typical crisis disorganization in the social and personality functioning of the parents and reflects the inadequacy of parents to cope with the new situation. Parents describe their own typical crisis reactions as follows: "It was as if my child had died. First, you go into shock, grieve; and then you gradually get over it." A father stated, "It seemed as if the world had come to an end." Gradually, he began to think of, "what was positive and what I could do for the child."

The need for providing short-term supportive counseling at the point of diagnostic impact, giving skilled anticipatory guidance over time, involving significant others and relevant agencies, and facilitating self-help support systems are all spotlighted by the crisis perspective of PKU.

RESPONSES TO THE DIAGNOSIS

Although there are variations, most parents react to the diagnosis with great intensity. "I feel doomed," is the way one mother expressed her response. A father had latent conflicts about sex and aggression come into awareness when the diagnosis reactivated a childhood memory in which he had witnessed the lynching of a neighbor who had raped a retarded child. This father developed a severe anxiety state which interfered with his work and other activities. Another parent went "berserk," became hysterical, and drove wildly on the freeway hoping that she would be killed. General worry and anxiety appear to characterize the reactions of most parents (Wood, *et al.*, 1967; Schild, 1968).

Another common reaction is depression. Parents frequently express feelings of despair, of, "Why has this happened to us?" and of great hurt and sadness for themselves and their child. In some instances, the depression is masked by avoidance and denial. The author knows of one couple who said they were going along with the medical treatment *only* to prove the diagnosis was in error. In another case, the paternal grandfather, a physician, would not accept that his son had to be a carrier for PKU. He projected the cause of the disease as due to his daughter-in-law, whom he did not relish. He instructed her to give Lofenalac to the child *only* when the PKU symptoms, such as exzema or hyperactivity became worse, thus treating isolated symptoms as they arose rather than thinking in terms of taking preventative measures.

The fact that PKU is genetically determined can be troubling to parents, particularly in relation to the conflicts surrounding further child bearing. Since the advent of newborn screening and the development of dietary therapy, PKU tends to be viewed as a disorder of high risk and low burden and, as a result, parents tend to be less conflicted about limiting family size (Leonard, *et al.*, 1972). Given the opportunity, parents are very willing to ventilate feelings about the impact of the genetic information on their lives, especially relative to family planning concerns.

The reactions of parents whose children are diagnosed beyond the newborn period differ from those whose infants are identified at birth. The former group of parents have noted with concern the slow development and/or behavioral problems of their children and have fears that mental retardation is present. Uncertainty and worry have already contaminated the parent–child relationship. Typically, these parents tend to become defensive and overprotective. They tend to project their hostility onto physicians, especially if they have made the rounds seeking answers regarding the child's difficulties. These parents tend to show more unreasoned personal guilt and greater preoccupation with the issue of mental retardation. Feelings of shame, stigma, and of difference, more akin to the larger population of parents of mentally retarded children tend to characterize these parents.

Among parents of newly diagnosed infants, relatively greater shock and bewilderment is seen due to the suddenness and unexpectedness of the diagnosis in seemingly normal infants. Depressive reactions are more common among mothers of children diagnosed at birth than among those of older diagnosed children. The grief of mothers of infants diagnosed with PKU at birth resembles that of mothers of defective children (Solnit & Stark, 1961). The early diagnosis takes on an illusive, somewhat nebulous quality, as the parents watch the treated newborn PKU child grow and thrive without apparent pathology. The parents operate under a constant threat that if they fail in maintaining the diet, their child will become brain damaged. They tend to respond with excessive monitoring and rigid management of the diet. In contrast to parents of later diagnosed children, they do not identify themselves as parents of mentally retarded children and have no stake in the social problem of mental retardation.

Regardless of the age at diagnosis, all parents are concerned about the length of time the child will need to remain on the diet and such future prospects as special schooling, employability, marriage, etc. Uncertainty about the future appears to underlie the visible distressful response of parents to the diagnosis (Tizard & Grad, 1961; Schild, 1968).

ADAPTATION TO THE DIETARY TREATMENT

Despite the negative attitudes parents generally have about the diet as drab, monotonous, and unappetizing, most families are able to adjust to the dietary treatment (Schild, 1964a; 1968.) The frequent serum phenylalanine testing and the inherent threat of possible brain damage act as potent motivating forces to adhere to the diet. Most parents report few problems with the diet; except with very young offspring. The siblings learn the diet and, usually, help to supervise the dietary regime. "Eating out" tends to be limited for an initial period following the initiation of the diet. Soon, however, families learn to cope with this minor problem. Parents tend to educate their neighbors, friends, and relatives about the disorder to discourage them from giving forbidden foods to the child. The main problem experienced is "snitching" of foods by the child, usually when the child is a toddler.

Parents generally are able to interpret the diet to the child readily and help the child to take responsibility for his own dietary control. The usual explanation given is that the child will become ill if he or she eats improper foods. The process is assisted by the concomitant routine medical check-ups that the child experiences.

Parents often feel guilty about depriving their children of special treats such as birthday cakes, ice cream, and so on, that their unaffected children may have. Expectedly, parents often react by indulging the child. This may interfere with other areas of child management such as in discipline. As the child becomes older and more independent, parents tend to have diminished tolerance for maintaining close dietary controls. As the diet is a constant reminder of the deviancy in the family, easing up on the rigors of maintaining the diet comes as a welcome relief.

Summary—Issues in Genetic Counseling

The diagnosis of PKU is a critical event for families which creates concerns about the affected member and generates various stresses on the total family unit. How the family adapts to the situation depends in great measure on how well they are initially counseled in regard to the genetic information and its implications. The genetic counselor must be sensitively attuned to the fact that the genetic diagnostic impact is unusually traumatic and disorganizing for the parents.

Dilemmas exist in some areas of genetic counseling with PKU families. Until a test for carrier determination of the individual case is developed, the provision of recurrence risks to siblings and extended relatives of the PKU individual will need to be made cautiously. Counseling PKU women about their reproductive risks of having mentally retarded offspring brings into sharp focus the ethical issues concerning the conflict between the right of the individual to free choice and the right of society to prevent, or at the very least, to recommend explicitly the prevention, of the birth of severely defective members. In the ethical context of contemporary genetic counseling, each counselor has to arrive at their own decision. Abiding by this principle may not, however, always feel comfortable to genetic counselors who are biased in the direction of societal responsibility and preventing genetic disease.

Another important problem is the need to make an accurate diagnosis of PKU to avoid giving erroneous genetic information and counsel to cases of hyperphenylalaninemia variants. Our ability to provide recurrence risks for such cases is currently limited.

The impact of the genetic information on marital and sexual relationships needs to be taken into account. Also, the family planning dilemmas which are evoked by the information require attention. It is doubtful that genetic counselors can provide the follow-up support services that families require to deal with these and other problems. For this reason, the issue of how to and who shall provide these supportive services needs to be considered. In some centers, PKU clinics have multidisciplinary staff including physicians, geneticists, nutritionists, public health nurses, and social workers available to provide this support. But in many locations, these centers do not exist or are not available or accessible. Who is to help when the PKU child is off the diet and no longer comes to the center for dietary supervision? The benefits of effective initial counseling may be greatly diminished if follow-up services are not provided. It is also important to be aware of the possibility that follow-up supportive work may not be able to easily undo the inadequacy of psychological support at the time of initial counseling.

More study needs to be made of how families cope with PKU. The limited research in this area suggests that, in general, parents have marked difficulty in making adequate adaptations to the problem, regardless of the stability of functioning prior to the time of diagnosis. A series of questions might be raised about the influence of the parents' inadequate adaptations on the patient, on each other, and on other family members. What are the possible disturbances engendered by PKU between the parent and patient and between the patient and siblings? How does the inadequacy of the parental adjustment to PKU influence family functioning and the vulnerability to subsequent life stresses? And, perhaps the most important question, in what ways can genetic counseling be enhanced so as to minimize the impact of the genetic disorder of PKU on the family members?

Case Illustrations

The R. Family
AN ILLUSTRATION OF INADEQUATE ADAPTATION TO THE PROBLEM OF PKU

The family consists of the parents, in their early 40s, and their three children. The youngest child was diagnosed as having PKU at 6 months of age. Mr. R. is an exceptionally bright man who has good technical employment but who has not achieved up to his intellectual ability. His wife is also of bright intelligence although she has not completed a high school education. Mrs. R. had a prior marriage; the eldest child in the family is a result of that union. The present marital relationship is warm and strong. Mr. R. has adopted his wife's child and shows no marked preferences for his own children.

The family lives in an attractive middle-class neighborhood in a relatively new, comfortably furnished four bedroom home. Living in the home also is Mrs. R's elderly grandfather who is alert mentally but who has several serious chronic health problems.

The two eldest sibs are intellectually gifted; one has an IQ score of 141 and the other an IQ of 133. These children are well-behaved and well-adjusted and are extremely gratifying to their parents.

The patient was compared from birth to her sibs. The parents were aware of her lethargy and lack of "exploratory interest" but denied that any basic slowness was present. When the diagnosis of PKU was made, Mrs. R. reacted with shock and great dismay. Mr. R. took a "scientific" attitude but like his wife resorted to considerable denial of the problem. He believed that something would be discovered to cure the child. For a long time, both parents resisted acknowledging the child's apparent mental retardation. They have become authoritative on every lay and scientific article written about the disorder. They pay particular heed to hints at cures or to doubts cast on the efficacy of the diet.

Since the parents have been unable to work through their feelings about the retardation, they are confused and inconsistent in their relationships with the child. They are overprotective, concerned, angry, and frustrated with her. Mrs. R. has found it difficult to adhere to the diet and needs to indulge the child in a compensatory way. The patient is mildly retarded ($IQ = 66$) and has considerable potential. However, this is being jeopardized by the inconsistent parenting.

Home has become a nightmare due to the irritability, hyperactivity, screaming, tantrum-like behavior of the child. During meals, the patient screams, demands attention, and makes conversation between family members impossible. The parents have been unable to sleep without interruption until recently when Mr. R. constructed a large locked play-pen type crib to keep the child in her room. Mrs. R. supervises the child's every waking minute. Privacy and free communication between family members is next to impossible when the child is awake. The family's social life has been drastically curtailed as it is difficult to take the patient anywhere or to find someone to care for her.

The parents have been very critical of the clinic. They have maintained a relationship with their private pediatrician and manipulate the medical advice of both sources as it suits their needs. They constantly question the validity of keeping the child on the diet. Mrs. R. feels she is depriving the child of adequate nourishment while Mr. R. has positive scientific proof that the diet is of little value. Although they claim to hold closely to the diet, all indications suggest that they have trouble doing so out of their inability to control the patient's behavior and their ambivalence about the value of the diet. They have no insight into how they have projected their feelings about the child onto the diet.

The parents have asked for help with their child but this has always been displaced onto concerns about the diet. The professionals working with this family have been trapped by the intellectualizations, rationalizations, and projections of these parents into focusing inappropriately on the diet.

The R's need help with their underlying feelings about having a deviant child. Meanwhile, they have progressively reinforced their inadequate defenses to the point where they have become more and more isolated from reality.

The M. Family
AN ILLUSTRATION OF ADEQUATE ADAPTATION TO THE PROBLEM OF PKU

This family consists of a Catholic couple with five children. The parents are college graduates and have been married for 12 years. They live in a modest home in a lower middle-class neighborhood. They are an attractive friendly couple who relate well to people and who have strong affectional, marital, and family bonds.

Prior to the diagnosis, the family lived in Canada. The early years of marriage were complicated by the scarcity of adequate employment in the father's profession and the mother's difficulties in childbearing. In the first 6 years of marriage, Mrs. M. was pregnant six times resulting in three live births, two miscarriages, and one child who died immediately after birth with hyaline membrane disease. The diagnosis of PKU was made on the second child when he was 23 months of age. At that time, the third child was also found to have PKU.

The family moved to California following the diagnosis on the advice of friends. Since that time Mr. M. has been steadily employed. They purchased a home, and two more (non-PKU) children were born. The two PKU patients have been under care at the clinic for the past 5 years.

The parents had a marked reaction to the diagnosis. Mr. M. has been able to verbalize the assault to his self-esteem; the feelings the diagnosis raised in reference to his virility and masculine ego. The parents were thrown into conflict about having further children in the face of the diagnosis and the mother's medical history. In addition to childbearing problems, Mrs. M. suffered from a kidney disorder that, at times, was life-threatening. The parents sought counsel with their priests and doctors, receiving conflicting advice. Ultimately, they were able to reconcile their devout Catholic beliefs with the reality of the health and genetic problems. This was no easy decision to make. At first, Mrs. M. used birth control. Subsequently, on medical advice, she had a hysterectomy.

The M's leaned on the clinic for help not only with the dietary care but for counsel on their personal concerns, for educational guidance, and for assistance with the financial problems created by the cost of the diet.

Over the 5 years that the children have been on the diet, the parents made an excellent adjustment to their life situation. They became active participants in their local community, taking an interest in neighbors, school system, local resources, and community problems. They accepted the fact that the diagnosis was made after the children had suffered some brain damage and realistically appraised the level of slowness in each child. They have worked closely with the local parent-group association for retarded children where their children were enrolled in nursery school. The M's provide the same cooperation to the public school where the boys are currently enrolled in special classes.

The M's are intelligent, perceptive parents who individualize the needs of their children. They are sensitive to the feelings of their eldest daughter who has recently been upset when neighborhood children referred to her brother as a "big retarded ape." The M's are empathetically trying to help their daughter cope with the reality aspects of the situation.

The parents have been helped considerably by the clinic staff. They were active participants in the group for PKU parents over a period of 2 years (Schild, 1964b). They found the group experience to be particularly helpful in working through feelings about the problem.

Currently, the M's are concerned with the exacerbation of the mother's kidney problem. This has forced them to consider an alternate plan for the elder PKU son who is moderately retarded and an extremely hyperactive child. He has become a behavior problem in the home. Though contemplating the possibility of state hospital placement, the M's showed normal ambivalence and guilt about this thinking. They hope to do the best for the child but realistically the M's are seeking solutions for the over-all family problem. With limited income, five children, a serious health problem of the mother, the M's are under considerable stress. They fear that their retarded son may become the target for their present tensions. The M's are purposefully seeking help with their present concerns and are showing caution and prudence in seeking a solution.

Despite the number of stresses this family has had to deal with, the parents have managed to cope fairly well with each crisis. The M's give the impression of being emotionally stable, and their children appear health, happy, and well-behaved. The family exudes an atmosphere of good mental health and optimism about the future.

SUMMARY OF CASE ILLUSTRATIONS

In contrasting the nature of the adaptations made by the two families, the essential factor appeared to be the way in which the parents were able to cope with the reactions which were evoked by the diagnosis. Despite their above average intelligence, and better economic security, the R. parents were apparently unable to handle their feelings about the personal meaning of the diagnosis. One might speculate that the diagnosis was a blow to their self-esteem and that they felt guilt and shame about the genetic defect. They attempted to handle their emotional reactions first by denial and projection. As time passed, their inability to resolve their negative feelings about the diagnosis became expressed in withdrawal from social contact, overprotectiveness of the child, and in unrealistic approaches to coping with the problems presented by the child. Their defensive denial colored their relationships with medical personnel and resulted in unrealistic hopes for a medical cure. They used intellectualization and rationalization to avoid dealing with the basic emotional conflicts stirred up by the diagnosis.

The M. family, on the other hand, despite the many serious problems that confronted them in their family life, were able to deal realistically with their emotional reactions to the diagnosis. Contrasted with the R. parents who had a history of difficulties in a previous marriage and failure in not achieving their full educational and occupational potential, the M. parents both showed successes in these areas.

The M's were both people with secure personalities and were able to acknowledge the negative feelings evoked by the diagnosis without threat to their self-image. They used the help offered to them over the years to strengthen their own capacities to cope with the difficult task of raising their PKU children. Rather than encapsulating themselves in self-pity and withdrawal from others, the M's sought support and comfort from relatives, friends, and professional people. They were cognizant of the needs of their normal children and attempted to see all of their children in perspective in their roles as family members.

Whereas the M. family managed to deal realistically with each new problem evoked by the diagnosis of PKU, the unrealistic approach of the R. family led them to an even more overwhelming situation than the one precipitated by the original diagnosis.

References

Acosta, P. B., Schaeffler, G. E., Wenz, E., & Koch, R. *PKU—A guide to management.* California State Department of Health, 1972.

Arthur, L. J. H. & Hulme, J. D. Intelligent small for dates born to oligophrenic phenylketonuric mothers after low-phenylalanine diets during pregnancy. *Pediatrics,* 1970, 46, 235.

Dobson, J. C., Kushida, E., Williamson, M., & Friedman, E. G. Intellectual performance of 36 PKU patients and their non-affected siblings. Unpublished paper, (undated).

Friedman, C. J., Sibinga, M. S., Steisel, I. M., & Sinnamon, H. A. Sensory restriction and isolation experiences in children with phenylketonuria. *Journal Abnormal Psychology,* 1968, 73, 294–303.

Koch, R., Blaskovics, M., Wenz, E., Fishler, K., & Schaeffler, G. Phenylalaninemia and phenylketonuria. In L. Nyhan, (Ed.). *Heritable Disorders of Amino Acid Metabolism*. N.Y.: Wiley and Sons, 1974.

Leonard, C. O., Chase, G. A., & Childs, B. Genetic counseling: A consumer's view. *New England Journal of Medicine*, 1972, 287, 433–439.

MacCready, R. A. & Levy, H. L. The problem of maternal phenylketonuria. *American Journal of Obstetrics & Gynecology*, 1971, 113, 131.

Mabry, C. C., Denniston, J. C., & Caldwell, J. A. A cause of mental retardation in children without metabolic defect. *New England Journal of Medicine*, 1963, 269, 1404.

President's Committee on Mental Retardation. *Mental retardation: The known and the unknown*. DHEW Publication (OHD), 76–21008, 1976.

Schild, Sylvia. Family attitudes and the low-phenylalanine diet. In *The clinical team looks at phenylketonuria*. HEW Washington, D.C. Government Printing Office, 1961., revised 1964a.

Schild, Sylvia. Parents of children with phenylketonuria. *Children*, 1964b, 2, 92–96.

Schild, Sylvia. Parental Adaptation to Phenylketonuria. Unpublished Doctoral Dissertation, School of Social Work, University of Southern California, Los Angeles, California, 1968.

Shear, C. S., Willman, N. S., & Nyhan, W. L. Phenylketonuria: Experience with diet and management. In W. L. Nyhan (Ed.). *Heritable disorders of amino acid metabolism*. New York: Wiley and Sons, 1974.

Sibinga, M. S. & Friedman, C. J. Complexities of parental understanding of phenylketonuria. *Pediatrics*, 1971, 48, 216–224.

Solnit, A. J. & Stark, M. H. Mourning and the birth of a defective child. *Psychoanalytic Study of the Child*. 1961, 16, 523–537.

Steisel, I. M., Friedman, C. J., & Wood, A. C. Interaction patterns in children with phenylketonuria. *Journal of Consulting Psychology*, 1967, 31, 162–168.

Steisel, J. M., Katz, K. S., & Harris, S. L. Controlling behavior of mothers of children with PKU. *Proceedings*, Collaborative Study of Children Treated for Phenylketonuria. 6th Nutritionists Conf. Aspen Colorado, p. 42–46, 1974.

Tizard, J. & Grad, J. C. *The mentally handicapped and their families: A social survey*. London: Oxford Press, 1961.

Wood, A. C., Friedman, C. J., & Steisel, I. M. Psychosocial factors in phenulketonuria. *American Journal of Orthopsychiatry*, 1967, 37, 671–679.

Psychological Issues in the Genetic Counseling of Cystic Fibrosis

9

Stanley E. Fischman

Cystic Fibrosis (CF) is an autosomal recessive disorder invariably manifesting itself in early life. The disorder affects multiple organ systems (lungs, liver, pancreas, gonads, etc.) and involves the mucous secreting glands of these organs as well as the electrolyte concentration of the sweat glands. The nature of the basic molecular defect of CF is unclear and diagnostic tests for the heterozygous state and/or fetal disease have not, as yet, been conclusively established.

CF occurs mostly among Caucasians. In fact, it is the most common lethal or semi-lethal genetic disease of Caucasians; its occurrence among Blacks and Orientals is unusual. The estimated frequency of heterozygotes in the Caucasian population is 1 in 20, with an estimated incidence of the disease (homozygote state) of 1 in 1500 to 1 in 2500 live births (di Sant'Agnese & Davis, 1976). The devastating effects of this genetic disorder on the individual, the parents and sibs, and on society at large should make CF a major concern not only to the medical world but to the greater community as well.

Clinical Aspects

The diagnosis of CF is usually established within the first few years of life. The earliest clinical manifestations of the disorder are generally pulmonary, although other abnormalities, such as meconeum ileus at birth or a fatty stool during infancy, may also lead to early diagnosis. The diagnosis needs to be confirmed by the Sweat Test, involving the

153

GENETIC COUNSELING
Psychological Dimensions

measurement of sweat electrolytes under controlled conditions; this test is considered pathognomonic of the disorder.

The major clinical problems of CF involve pulmonary infections and progressive destruction of lung parenchyma secondary to the production of a very thick and tenacious sputum. The subsequent obstruction of the bronchial tree by this abnormal sputum leads to the formation of the lung cysts from which the disorder derives its name. In addition, affected individuals are unable to adequately absorb foodstuffs from their intestines due to the disturbances within the enzyme secreting (exocrine) glands of the pancreas and liver. This paucity of enzyme production also leads to a progressive destruction of these organs, often eventuating in the further complications of diabetes and/or hepatic cirrhosis.

Until recent years, the vast majority of affected children did not survive the early teenage period; many died within the first few years of life. Improvements in medical treatment, which include the chronic administration of antibiotics, oral enzymes, and appropriate salt replacement as well as the use of technical and physical aids in pulmonary toileting, have greatly increased the chance of an affected child living into the teen years and even adulthood.

In the discussion that follows, I plan to consider some of the emotional consequences of CF for the affected person. Initially, the focus will be on the symptomatic problems associated with the respiratory and gastrointestinal systems and the ensuing disturbances of the individual's body image. Then the social problems commonly associated with the occurrence of CF will be considered. The responses of the parents, of the healthy siblings, and of the affected individuals surviving into adulthood will be considered in turn. Finally, some of the counseling and psychotherapeutic issues of CF will be discussed.

Emotional Issues

The symptoms of CF rather than the notion of the disease per se often have a profound impact on the affected child's emotional development. Many clinical symptoms arise as a result of the involvement of the mucous secretory and the gastrointestinal systems. These symptoms lead to major psychological and social problems in addition to the physical difficulties involved.

RESPIRATORY SYSTEM

The patients endure repeated hospitalizations both for recurrent pneumonia as well as prophylactic pulmonary toileting. During these hospitalizations, family life is disrupted and the youngster often is confronted with having to fall behind peers in school, athletics and social life. In our clinical experience, this is a major concern for the child during the pre-adolescent and early pubertal years. This is the period of development, described by Erikson, in which children form their sense of personal competence, their body images, and their images of potential adult functioning.

To make matters worse, the progressive failure of the respiratory system leads to increasing shortness of breath and decreasing stamina, so that the children with CF increasingly find themselves falling behind their peers just as the other children are becoming increasingly engaged in more rugged activities. The CF child may become isolated, withdrawn, develop a "school phobia," and/or many exaggerated or factitious symptoms to avoid being rejected by peers. Coping with the disorder through school avoidance is particularly prominent in the early teenager.

The hacking cough and the thickened, foul-smelling sputum also affect the patient's interaction with peers. At best, most others find the cough annoying; at worst, loathsome. Even after repeated reassurance to the contrary, peers and their parents fear that the "disease" is contagious and that it might be a variant of tuberculosis. This latter notion is reinforced by the frail and cachectic appearance of many children with CF, a major factor in the development of a poor body image in these individuals.

GASTROINTESTINAL SYSTEM

One of the symptoms involving this system with a particular emotional relevance is the production of a fatty, foul-smelling stool and the frequent passage of flatus, despite the utilization of oral enzyme replacement. This is usually a source of considerable embarrassment to the young adult or child with CF. Our experience with young adolescents (ages 13–15) in activity groups suggests that this one symptom by itself exacts a heavy emotional toll. Once relaxed, the members of such groups banter and "joke" about the odor of each other's feces and continually mimic "farting" noises with their lips or balloons. Often this latter behavior is a prelude to serious discussions of the issue of embarrassment, of concerns about their physical vulnerability and "incompleteness," and of fears regarding their acceptability to normal peers and members of the opposite sex.

BODY IMAGE

One of the normal critical developmental tasks of adolescence is the reformulation and consolidation of the person's body image. It is easy to imagine how CF would impact on this task. The problems of these patients often involve a small size, a disproportionate growth of the chest to compensate for compromised lung function ("barrel-chest"), a protuberant abdomen, delayed sexual maturation and development, and clubbing of the fingertips. Some of the common strategies used to cope with these problems include avoidance and overcompensation. The patients may refuse to attend school and/or become severely withdrawn; some, on the other hand, attempt to push themselves to the limits of their physical capacities and/or perpetrate acts of bravado. Because these strategies are directed toward avoiding or denying stage-specific tasks, they often lead to further developmental difficulties.

Another major area of concern for every young person emerging into adulthood involves issues of dependence and independence. The presence of the illness precludes an easy transition from adolescence to adulthood since it renders the affected person dependent, to greater or lesser degree, on parents, medication and equipment, medical personnel, and hospitals. To achieve a sense of independence, the young person may engage in rebellion or oppositional behavior. Treatments, especially unpleasant ones or those that disrupt "important" activities and reflect dependence on others (e.g., percussion and drainage), are often refused.

Denial appears to be the principal coping strategy used to deal with the impairment of the body construct as well as the issue of dependency. In refusing necessary medications or by engaging in sports activities that overextend the physical capacities of the CF individual, the victim is acting as if the disease was not present. Interestingly, in my experience, behaviors suggestive of denial appear more frequently in youngsters who have a relative paucity of external manifestations of the disease; it is probably easier to deny the illness in these cases.

As the affected individual strives for greater independence, concerns increase regarding the question of who will provide the life-sustaining care formerly given by parents and significant others. Thus, in contrast to the normal person, where steps toward greater independence are often associated with a growing sense of competence and mastery, those of the individual with CF may increase the sense of insecurity and thoughts of mortality (Tropauer, Franz, & Dilgard, 1970).

Social Considerations

Possibly the greatest psychosocial impact of CF involves the interdependence which develops between parents and patient as a result of the illness and its treatment plan. The constant monitoring for early signs of illness, the percussion treatment at home (often required as much as four times a day), and the need to monitor a large number of medications for the affected child often interfere with the natural processes of individuation and growth into independent adulthood. In addition, the parents' own fears regarding this disorder may impede their ability to share their feelings and thoughts and otherwise communicate with each other, the patient, and other sibs. When communication difficulties predominate, psychological distortions of the relationships within the family increasingly develop, and, often, interfere with the medical management of the disorder.

PARENTAL RESPONSES

Prior to the confirmation of the diagnosis of CF, most parents are already suspicious that there is something seriously "wrong" with their child. However, because of the common nature of the presenting symptoms (respiratory infections, diarrhea), the physician often overlooks the diagnosis until the symptoms become so persistent or so debilitating that the appropriate diagnostic work-up is pursued.

Parents react to the diagnosis of CF as they might to any potentially devastating illness (e.g., cancer, serious mental retardation) and experience shock, denial, and depression as they grapple with their feelings of guilt, anger, sadness, and fear as well as their feelings of inadequacy and loss. The fact that CF is genetically based can either exacerbate or mitigate some of these emotional responses.

There is a critical need for medical personnel to appreciate and recognize the various psychological processes that the parents are experiencing; these impede parental ability to accurately absorb the information concerning the nature of their child's illness and the treatment program. Many of the processes involved in the *normal* coping response such as *shock* and *denial* require that information be screened, distorted, and obfuscated, usually in the service of protecting the ego (i.e., coping). Unfortunately, these processes are often perceived by medical personnel as signs of weakness or of impending disintegration and annoyed or fearful responses are sometimes evoked. Even stronger opprobrium of medical personnel is evoked when the parents display depression or hostility. These latter affects usually occur after some time has passed following the establishment of the diagnosis; they reflect the gradual acceptance of the devastating nature of the disease and of the tasks that lie ahead.

Hostility is particularly difficult for caretakers to accept, especially in the face of their own feelings of relative helplessness and given the amount of energy they have expended in the care of the child and his family. In the absence of an understanding of the coping dynamics underlying the parents' hostility, the natural response is to view them as ungrateful, uncooperative, and unreasonable. This reaction, of course, may lead to a further breakdown in the relationship between the professional and the parents and, eventually, to a more realistic basis for mutual distrust. If the hostile reaction can be understood as a transient, perhaps appropriate step in coping with intolerable reality, and *not* as a personal attack on the health professional, a positive relationship may emerge and the parents' acceptance of the disorder may be facilitated. It is not unusual to hear parents, well along in the successful acceptance of the reality of the disease, to reflect on these episodes with their physician and to express their gratefulness that he or she allowed them to "take out their feelings" on him or her at the time.

On the home front, the practical burdens placed on the parents of children with CF are enormous and include major financial pressures (even when direct medical and hospitalization costs are assumed by insurance companies and/or governmental sources), the interruption of career and other family goals, and the disruption of daily routines because of home treatments, repeated hospitalizations, and clinic visits.

Parents also experience numerous changes in their relationships with other adults and families. They become increasingly isolated from simple, mundane activities with other families because of the limitations imposed by the treatments of the disease required to be carried out in the home. Their personal sense of isolation and disruption are usually increased during periods of illness and hospitalizations of the child. Parents frequently experience enormous guilt over the possibility that they have not done enough or given of themselves sufficiently to the affected child. Thus, they blame themselves for exacerbations of the illness or for the relapses requiring hospitalization. This leads to further escalations of the "doing" phenomenon described in other CF families (Leiken & Hassakis, 1973).

To compound the parents' problems in these areas, other adults tend to avoid them because of their own anxieties about "facing them." It is not unusual for a parent to report that people "cross the street" rather than meet up with them.

The question of further pregnancies is a major burden in situations in which the diagnosis is made early in the development of the family. Given that the recurrence risk is one in four and that no definitive test for antenatal diagnosis is available, the decision invariably generates trepidation and misgiving. There is a wide spectrum of responses to further childbearing even in relatively well functioning CF families. One unusual family with which I have had extensive contact, had five affected children out of eight! They have firm convictions that their decision to continue to have children was justified. Both of these parents have been very involved and concerned with all of their children and the three children with CF who have lived into their teens have been happy, active, and involved people. One daughter, who recently died, was a source of great inspiration to a number of other children with CF and other chronic diseases. Interestingly, this family has had to bear considerable criticism from health professionals as well as other CF families for having brought so many affected children into this world.[1]

RESPONSES OF UNAFFECTED SIBS

Little has been written about the unaffected sibs of CF individuals even though they face many unusual stresses as a result of having a brother or sister with CF. Besides the obvious problems associated with the loss of personal attention due to the focus on the ill sib and the interruption of normal family activities and pursuits, the healthy child faces problems resulting from inconsistent parenting, guilt, depression, and uncertainties about the future.

Especially in adolescence and young adulthood, healthy sibs often express concerns that their affected sister or brother tends to be "spoiled" or overprotected by their parents. While this is a justifiable assessment, there is a clear tendency for parents to also "overprotect" the well sibs, particularly after the death of an affected sib. This often results in an over-reaction to somatic complaints by both the sib and the parents. Psychosomatic illness as well as school avoidance symptoms (headache, abdominal pain, malaise) are prominent in the sibs of many patients with chronic and debilitating illnesses.

Sibs, when young, often imagine that they have "caused" the periodic exacerbations of clinical symptoms or even the illness itself. They harbor guilt feelings over their unconscious wishes and conscious resentments. These sometimes return to haunt them, especially after the death of the sib.

Another issue which seems to engender sibling guilt is the counterpoint of the familiar question, "Why me?", which is rhetorically asked when we become seriously ill. In this case the unaffected sibs often utilize fantasies about past behavior and/or secret powers to explain why they were spared, particularly as the glimmerings of the genetic nature of the illness enter their understanding—in effect, trying to answer the question, "Why *not* me?"

On the social level, many unaffected sibs report having to deal with rejection on the part of peers and adults because of their fears of contagion

---

[1] This should not be taken as endorsement of reproduction in families at risk for further CF children. I merely want to stress the necessity for greater understanding of the needs of such families on the part of health professionals.

or, on a more subtle level, because of their difficulties in controlling their feelings or "saying the wrong thing" to the sib, and hurting his or her feelings. Thus, in an effort to be solicitous and protective, many individuals isolate and reject the sibs of CF persons.

The fact that the unaffected sib may possess a deleterious gene may also present problems during normal adolescence and around the time of marriage. During adolescence, the sense of somehow being defective or incomplete often leads to vague and haunting feelings of inadequacy, which, in turn, frequently interferes with the development of an adequate self-image in the teenager. Serious behavioral difficulties may result (delinquency, depression, overwhelming "free-floating" anxiety). On the other hand, these concerns over one's adequacy may be channeled into powerfully productive pursuits and be a directing force during the periods of uncertainty which often plague normal adolescents.

When marriage is contemplated, the feelings of inadequacy or defectiveness can interfere with the decision to commit oneself to a binding relationship with another human being. In addition, nagging fears of potential damage to yet unborn children may cloud the relationship between the unaffected sib and the spouse. These fears do not appear to mitigate with time and marital success; indeed, they seem to recur with each pregnancy. Perhaps this painful, nagging experience will be ameliorated in some individuals when adequate tests for the heterozygote state and/or the presence of CF *in utero* are perfected.

AFFECTED INDIVIDUALS IN ADULTHOOD

A special group that merits discussion is the ever increasing number of affected individuals who are living into adulthood, holding full and part-time jobs and leading lives independent of their nuclear families. These individuals find themselves in a unique position, since survival into adulthood was considered science-fiction only a few years ago. We now see many patients who are nurses, respiratory therapists, journalists, college students, and industrial workers. Many have married and a few have had children of their own. Although the CF male is usually sterile, some have become fathers through artificial insemination techniques. These developments raise a number of moral and ethical questions, which will probably be debated vehemently over the next few years.

There are also some practical problems which this group frequently needs to face. For instance, specialists in adult diseases often are uncomfortable treating them, and even when the patients are in their 30s, medical care continues to be rendered by pediatricians, often based in hospitals or clinics established for children. This can hardly have a positive effect on the person's self-esteem.

At work, they have to deal with the concerns of their co-workers about their health (the hacking cough and frail appearance are particularly consternating). Many adults with CF do not reveal the nature of their illness to co-workers for fear of being subjected to differential treatment or to actual job loss. Often they withhold information about the illness when they apply for jobs out of a concern about health insurance coverage; many CF adults believe that companies would refuse to hire them because they would have to pay higher insurance premiums for all their employees.

GENETIC COUNSELING ISSUES

In the course of providing recurrence risk information, it becomes important for counselors to distinguish between their own values and needs and those of the counselees. For example, the counselors may value highly the prevention of further cases of CF in a family, which, from their perspective, is already burdened, socially, psychologically, and financially with an affected individual. The counselors will be strongly tempted to assume that the family members will see and evaluate their predicament in the same way they do. Such assumptions on the part of the counselors may be widely off the mark and, unfortunately, because of a sense of courtesy, deference, or protocol, the counselees may not provide the counselors with correcting information. Under other circumstances, as for example, in psychotherapy, such discrepancies often emerge and the family member(s) have an opportunity to vent their resentments and the other feelings which were withheld from the genetic counselors.

As a routine part of the genetic counseling an exploration for unresolved feelings of guilt, resentment, etc. with the affected individual, spouse, and/or the family should be made. Also, family members should be helped to express their perspectives as to the effects of the disease on individual family members and on the family in general. If the parents of an affected child are the counselees, it might be determined how well the parents are managing financially and what difficulties they have encountered in their raising the affected child and other children, in their interpersonal relations, etc. If the child has died, the effect this has had on the spouses individually and on the family needs to be determined. At each step of the way, support of their efforts to cope with the disorder and its consequences is provided.

If an unaffected sib is the counselee, I generally ask them what it was like being the brother or sister of someone with CF and thus afford them an opportunity to express whatever it is they need to say on this subject. Old resentments and hurts may be revealed. It may often be helpful to ask if their past experiences were only negative ones, thus allowing them to experience other feelings they may have towards the affected sib—the caring and love, which, paradoxically, are often more difficult to express than are the anger and resentments. In one notable case that comes to mind, the sib of a CF individual who had died almost 15 years earlier, was able to verbalize that indeed there were also fun times together in the past and that she missed her dead brother. It is important to help the person see a fuller picture of what his or her life experiences with CF have been. When the person comes to realize that the affected individual's life was not wasted; that the life had meaning, that there was an impact on parents and sibs and possibly on others as well; that he or she left a mark rather than a scar on the world, then the person's own life and experiences take on a richer meaning and deeper significance.

In my experience, the genetic counseling of affected individuals frequently takes the form of strongly advising them not to have children. (Such tactics are consistent with the general tendency of medical personnel to infantalize the CF person as well as their parents.) This, generally, is counterproductive and undermines the individual's autonomy. It may be far better to explore with the counselees the meaning of having a child and the degree of reality-based thinking regarding what it might mean to raise a child, given the debilitating nature of the illness and the likelihood that the parents will not witness the maturation of the CF child.

Therapeutic Issues

Repeated studies and observations indicate that the various coping responses of patients, families, and professionals to CF have a major impact on both the physical *and* the emotional aspects of the illness. The differences in responses of those affected by CF are quite extreme. Some patients withdraw while others flourish and become inspirations for others, sick and healthy alike. Some families suffer breakdown on many fronts while others seem to tap an inner strength and provide succor to those in contact with them.

Most children with CF have their care coordinated through a hospital or clinic setting. This provides an opportunity to develop staff sensitivities as well as programs to assist the affected person to develop coping skills that enable him or her to make the most of life, however short it may be, and thus enhance the physical and emotional outcome. One of the major needs, with respect to staff sensitivities, is for a reframing of attitudes toward the so-called "problems" of CF individuals and their families. Perhaps it might be more appropriate to view many of these "problems" as coping responses and attempts at adaptation to a serious, chronic illness. So long as the behavior of the family members is viewed as oppositional and resistive or in some other negative light, the professional is fostering a system of antagonism and conflict between himself or herself and the family. This is unlikely to lead to positive relationships between the professional and the family and may interfere with the provision of optimal health care. One example of how such reframing might proceed is Self-Help groups. The efficacy of such groups has been demonstrated in a variety of situations, ranging from drug addiction to mastectomy. It is critical that Self-Help groups be organized for mutual support and be oriented toward activity and information-giving rather than being labeled as "therapy." The notion of a therapist ministering to the needs of the needy often is counterproductive as it undermines the self-esteem for which handicapped individuals so desperately strive. In fact, Self-Help groups are usually most effective when organized and managed by the affected individuals rather than by professionals. The latter can best provide help by assisting the leadership of the group to obtain technical support (space, funds, etc.) and official auspices and sanction to enable the group activities to occur (speakers, insurance, etc.).

I have had direct experience with such a CF group and the results have been most salutary. The group, organized by young adult patients with CF, provides unique informational sharing and personal support, as well as helpful changes within the hospital structure and medical program. Above all, the group provided its members with a strong sense of identification as well as of a feeling of "not being alone with the disease." The group has been so successful that it eventually attracted a number of patients who live as much as 100 miles away for evening meetings! An informative newsletter organized and published by this group has gained national prominence.

Similar groups have provided appropriate outlets and support systems for parents of children with CF. Hopefully, similar types of groups will develop for the unaffected sibs of patients.

A word of caution is in order here. Some parents have found themselves devoting too much energy and time to these organizations, often at the expense of the family. Sometimes, this excessive involvement reflects a temporary and futile attempt at coping with unresolved feelings about the child's illness. Professional counseling is generally indicated in such instances.

Other group approaches have been particularly useful to older adolescents and adults. The younger adolescent has special needs related to the normal psychological issues of that developmental period. Physical competence and social acceptability loom high on the priority scale for children at this age, and the youngster with CF must deal with the special disadvantages in this area. Towards this end, opportunities for specially designed cosmetic and physical conditioning programs, group activities emphasizing physical competence (e.g., survival training, camping), and simple tips for enhancing their attractiveness should be undertaken. The concerns over looking young, "short and skinny," and sexually immature are particularly troublesome and can be helped, to some degree, by appropriate grooming. Personnel involved in such activities with this age group need to be aware of the specific fears associated with the symptoms of CF and to be prepared to pursue these concerns in a supportive fashion when appropriate opportunities arise.

A recent incident illustrates this point: A 15-year-old boy who has physically fared relatively well with CF and had relatively little progression of his disease, had not been attending school for approximately 3 years. He frequently had vague but severe abdominal symptoms, occasionally requiring hospitalization because of persistent vomiting. Despite extensive evaluations, no physical basis for the pain and vomiting could be elucidated. As time progressed, it became clear that there was a large emotional component to his physical symptoms and it became apparent that we were dealing with a "school phobia." Appropriate testing revealed severe learning disabilities and, although reluctantly accepted by this youngster, attempts at remediation were begun. He began psychotherapy and while many strides were made in therapy, he still did not want to return to school and frustrated the many attempts made by cooperative school personnel to make that transition possible. Abruptly, he did return to school for no apparent reason and began to do quite well academically despite his "learning disabilities." On a CF camping trip, he mentioned the real reason offhandedly to one of the leaders: He had often found a greasy stain (secondary to the poor digestion of dietary fat) on the seat of his pants and was too embarrassed to appear in public. He finally discovered that wearing heavy denim pants tended to hide this stain and thus he could return to school. Further material emerged because the camping leader took advantage of the opportunity offered by the "confession" to engage the other adolescents with CF in a frank discussion of their fears and concerns in this area. Many of the young people had experienced similar grease stains and had been mortified when this was called to their attention by peers. A sharing of techniques to combat this problem followed. The sense of relief about openly discussing such a secretive matter and finding out they "were not alone" was very obvious.

Interestingly, since that time, some members of that camping group have become much more socially outgoing and assertive and also have taken an increased interest in following their therapeutic regimens.

Vocational help for the older patient and help in maintaining scholastic endeavors during the many hospitalizations are important for maintaining patient confidence and self-worth. Vocational help need not be provided entirely by professionals or by state agencies, which often have rules, regulations, and expectations inappropriate to the special needs of the patient with CF. Some of the most effective vocational counseling I have seen has been given by other patients with similar handicaps who *have* been successful at adult careers. Their very success conveys a powerful message.

To sum up, CF is a serious, multi-organ genetic disease that progressively handicaps its victims, physically and emotionally. Psychosocial problems appear largely related to the impact of the characteristic symptoms on normal developmental tasks. Family members are also burdened by the symptoms, the treatment demands, and the impending loss. Amelioration of some of the devastating effects can often be attained by strengthening individual and family coping processes. Especially useful are opportunities to develop an identification with others similarly affected and feelings of competency.

References

Bowman, B. H. and Mangos, J. A. Current concepts in genetics: Cystic fibrosis. *New England Journal of Medicine*, 1976, 294, 937–938.

di Sant'Agnese, P. A. & Davis, P. B. Research in cystic fibrosis. *New England Journal of Medicine*, 1976, 295, 481.

Leiken, S. J. & Hassakis, P. Psychological study of parents of children with cystic fibrosis. In E. J. Anthony and C. Koupernik (Eds.), *The Child in His Family*, Vol. 2. New York: John Wiley and Sons, 1973.

Tropauer, A., Franz, M. N. & Dilgard, V. W. Psychological aspects of the care of children with cystic fibrosis. *American Journal of Diseases of Children*, 1970, 119, 424–432.

Applied Behavioral Genetics: Counseling and Psychotherapy in Sex-Chromosomal Disorders

10

John Money,
Andrew Klein,
John Beck

In this chapter we will discuss three of the major sex chromosome abnormalities and the problems associated with them. We will focus on three syndromes: 45, X (Turner's), 47, XXY (Klinefelter's) and 47, XYY, using the approach termed applied behavioral cytogenetics (Money, 1975). We start with the premise that a better understanding of psychodynamics specific to the syndrome facilitates the individual case management of persons with these syndromes, and that it provides counselors with a base of information that they need in prospective genetic counseling or in the counseling of couples where these chromosomal disorders are detected in the course of amniocentesis and/or subsequent fetal karyotyping.

Turner's Syndrome

SIGNS AND SYMPTOMS

Turner's syndrome is a clinical condition which stems from a chromosomal anomaly. One chromosome of the sex chromosome pair is missing, the remaining one being always an X, so that the total is only 45 $(44 + X)$. Variations of this syndrome exist when the missing X chromosome is imperfectly represented as a fragmented chromosome, an isochromosome, or in a mosaic. The incidence of Turner's syndrome is 1:2500 live-born girls. The occurrence is sporadic and typically occurs only once in a family pedigree. There are no clues that might lead to an attempt at prenatal

167

GENETIC COUNSELING
Psychological Dimensions

diagnosis by means of amniocentesis, and there is no known form of prenatal intervention that would be effective in correcting the condition.

The two pathognomonic signs of Turner's syndrome are short stature in a person with the body morphology of a female and absence of the ovaries (gonadal agenesis or dysgenesis). The affected person is sterile and sexually infantile in appearance until hormonally treated. Other associated developmental anomalies have been described in this syndrome, all or any of which may or may not occur in a given individual. These anomalies include webbed neck, underdevelopment of the chin, epicanthal folds (resembling those of oriental eyes), shield-like chest, pigmented moles, kidney and heart defects, and hearing loss.

BEHAVIORAL CHARACTERISTICS

In addition to the cytogenetic and endocrinologic signs of Turner's syndrome, there are behavioral symptoms that frequently accompany the diagnosis. Included are deficits in space–form perception and directional sense, and motor clumsiness. There is also a personality feature which has been termed inertia of emotional arousal. This feature is marked by complacency, stolidity, and slowness in asserting initiative. Behaviorally, however, and possibly relating to this inertia of emotional arousal, females with Turner's syndrome have an unusual capacity to deal with stress and adversity. The prevalence of psychiatric disability is remarkably low. Psychosexually, the patients are the epitome of femininity and are maternal in their play and child care interests from infancy onward.

COUNSELING

Neuropsychologic studies of patients with Turner's syndrome have indicated on the basis of Wechsler Intelligence Scales and the Benton Visual Retention Test, among others, that many affected patients possess a specific cognitive defect in space-form perception (praxic reasoning). According to these findings, the Wechsler performance IQ in Turner's syndrome averages approximately 20 points lower than the verbal IQ. Thus an appearance of an increased incidence of slight mental retardation may in fact, be attributed to impairment of nonverbal ability only. Tasks that are included in the category of space-form disability are those that require accurate perception and logical manipulation of form and spatial properties of a stimulus. Thus, a Turner patient might have exceptional difficulty with such school tasks as map-reading, figure-drawing, geometry, and even arithmetic. These difficulties might require, in some cases, the counselor's intervention at the school, in order to explain the condition to the patient's teachers. Counseling the patient in this respect can best be accomplished by reinforcing the fact that her greatest academic and vocational strength lies in her verbal skill.

Some Turner patients exhibit a tendency towards motor clumsiness. In an extreme form this could also justify intervention on the part of the counselor. A letter written to the school recommending deletion of physical education from the patient's schedule has been proven beneficial. Such a letter also eliminates problems due to exposure of bodily deformities and early in teenage, delay of onset of breast development.

Money and Mittenthal in 1970 showed that parental rejection and parental psychopathology, and to a lesser extent overprotectiveness, are directly associated with psychopathology in the daughters with Turner's syndrome. Some patients must thus cope with parental pathology. The counselor or psychotherapist can be of benefit in aiding the patient in practicing healthy responses and in finding solutions to parent–child relationship problems.

Several of the stigmata of Turner's syndrome are of great personal psychologic significance. Thus, reference to these stigmata needs to be presented in a sensitive manner and geared to the age and understanding of the individual patient. It is tempting to avoid the topic of sterility under the guise of sparing the child or adolescent undue emotional trauma. Facial expressions and body language of physicians and parents, however, coupled with the medical interest in the genitalia during physical examinations will betray the presence of a sex-related problem. To prevent the inference of misinformation, the counselor needs to deal directly with the subject of sterility. An ideal way to disclose unpleasant medical predictions is to place them in the context of probability and the laws of chance. It is a cardinal principle in counseling that one never makes prophecies, but only actuarial predictions. The counselor can disclose the probability of sterility and indicate that it is expected that the patient can achieve motherhood by adoption. Stated in this positive fashion, the idea of parenthood remains intact. Only the means of achieving the end is altered. With this knowledge, the child can build the concept of motherhood by adoption, or by marrying an "instant family," rather than by pregnancy, into her fantasies concerning the future. So prepared, the girl has an increased chance for success in meeting her special role, and also of preparing her spouse in advance.

Girls with Turner's syndrome, because of their smallness and late onset of induced puberty (via hormone replacement), encounter many situations, episodic or continuous, of being treated as though they were immature. In counseling the patient's parents, it is essential to point out their own propensity to relate to the child in terms of her statural age rather than her chronological age. Another component of the counseling regimen is preparing the patient for the taunts of her peers and the condescending attitudes taken by ignorant others.

A recurrent problem in patients of short stature is that of their desire for socialization and their inability to find others equally short in stature. Two national organizations can aid in this task—Human Growth Incorporated and Little People of America. Association with others having similar difficulties can ameliorate a feeling of isolation and can aid a person in terms of sharing problems and solutions concerning statural deficit.

Because patients with Turner's syndrome exhibit behavior characterized by a high tolerance for adversity, they adapt to life more easily than might be expected considering the problems they face. It is possible that the genetic defect producing the adverse symptoms and stigmata of Turner's syndrome also produces a beneficial effect, that of increasing the person's tolerance of the syndrome's physical symptoms. Even though the prevalence of severe psychopathology has been low in the sample studied in our clinic, serious psychopathology has been noted. The following case illustrates both the shared and the unique biographical problems that can be related to the diagnosis of Turner's syndrome.

CASE ILLUSTRATION

Cindy S., a female with minimal stigmata of Turner's syndrome, was first seen at The Johns Hopkins Hospital and diagnosed as a Turner patient at the age of 10. She was referred to the psychohormonal research unit from the pediatric endocrine clinic because she was having severe psychologic difficulties associated with short stature. Since that time, for 8 years, she has been followed regularly in the psychohormonal research unit.

The patient exhibits some of the behavioral signs of Turner's syndrome, namely, a deficit in space–form reasoning, a degree of poor motor coordination, and clearly feminine and maternal interests. In addition to these, however, she exhibits several unique behavioral traits.

During her early teen years, for approximately 1 year, the patient was periodically obsessed with thoughts of suicide. The precipitating incident, disclosed only after an interval of 2 years, evolved from a betrayal of confidence by a friend concerning her medical condition. Males in her classroom used this information to tease her excessively, indicating that she would be a safe female for sexual experimentation, since pregnancy would be impossible. This teasing offended the patient to the point that she created for herself an alternative identity. She told her classmates one morning that she was her cousin and that the C.S. they knew had gone to Hollywood. She hoped this would have the effect of making her classmates like and accept her. In fact, it simply added to her burden the gossip that she might be crazy.

On other occasions the patient expressed interest in having facial plastic surgery. She indicated that she wanted a new personality and a new image. She thought she had had a reputation since elementary school for being a jerk or a dope. This she hoped to remedy by facial surgery, an idea borrowed from her mother's history.

Psychodynamically, the initial phenomenon of alternative identity corresponds to a diagnosis of multiple personality or dissociative reaction. The desire for cosmetic surgery illustrates the displacement of concern from a short stature and failed puberty problem to appearance of the face, which was alterable, but did not need alteration.

Gradually, with psychotherapy of a medical supportive nature, the suicidal thoughts subsided. The patient gradually understood the relation of her thoughts to her shortness and delayed onset of somatic puberty. She realized she was being treated socially in accordance with her height age rather than her chronological age. With the onset of estrogen treatment her pathologic behavior has lessened.

The patient is presently majoring in political science at a large state university. She is considering law as a future profession, but is concerned that she may not score adequately on the law school entrance exam owing to mathematical and space–form cognitional deficit (Verbal IQ 114; Performance IQ 89; Full IQ 104). Should that be the case, her application will be supported by a strong letter of explanation and endorsement from the psychohormonal research unit.

Despite a relative lack in social life, she was disinclined to attend meetings of a human-potential group for short people. It was more important to her to be accepted into a college sorority, irrespective of her height. She did, in fact, become a sorority sister and her social life made some improvement, evidenced in obvious progress in social maturity and self-esteem.

All things considered, it has been far from easy for this patient to cope with all the problems consequent on a missing chromosome. Without knowledge of the diagnosis and prognosis and appropriate counseling, it would have been all but impossible for her parents to be maximally effective in their dealings with their daughter, and for her doctors to provide help for her. It also would have been impossible for the girl herself to have been maximally expeditious in self-help.

Klinefelter's Syndrome

SIGNS AND SYMPTOMS

In contrast to Turner's syndrome which is characterized by a deficit in the amount of genetic material, Klinefelter's syndrome involves a supernumerary X chromosome. Patients with Klinefelter's syndrome commonly present the following somatic findings: small testes with aspermatogenesis, a small penis (borderline average or smaller), tall stature, gynecomastia, and sparse facial and sexual hair (sometimes with a feminine distribution). Unless a buccal smear is performed, one is unlikely to make a diagnosis of Klinefelter's syndrome in a prepubertal male. Buccal smears are not routinely employed for screening newborn infants. Thus the condition often remains covert until after the onset of puberty. Prevalence of the syndrome in newborn males has been estimated from neonatal screening studies at 1:500.

BEHAVIORAL CHARACTERISTICS

All the behavioral traits, excepting sporadically-occurring major psychiatric symptoms, that have been attributed to men with the XXY syndrome appear to be secondary to three basic conditions or characteristics of the syndrome: sexual apathy, easy fatiguability, and low dominance assertion. These three characteristics create an impression of what, in the older French literature, was called neurasthenia, and in the U.S. literature today is often referred to as inadequate personality.

All three characteristics may be seen as stemming possibly from a common origin in insensitivity or hyporesponsiveness of XXY cells to androgen. The basis of this statement lies in the well known clinical facts of the XXY syndrome at puberty, namely that the onset of puberty may be relatively tardy, and that adult virilization is typically below average or even inadequate.

Severe mental deficiency may be a concomitant of the 47, XXY syndrome, though the IQ may also be normal or superior. When the individual is mentally retarded, it is both the verbal and nonverbal intelligence which are affected, in contrast to Turner's syndrome, where the deficit lies in nonverbal intelligence specifically.

COUNSELING

A supernumerary X chromosome is likely to expose an individual to an impairment, deficiency, or inhibition of doing. With this concept in mind, the therapist should devise a counseling program which, while not nihilistic, is supportive when the patient is confronted with his inability to achieve on a par with his peers. Although the plasma testosterone levels of XXY men may be within normal range, in some patients, it is possible to get a positive response by injecting long-acting testosterone enanthate in an amount (300 or 400 mg every 4 weeks) sufficient to be slightly in excess of a replacement dosage for a castrate. The positive response is mild and is manifested as an increased frequency of erotic imagery and initiative, improved feelings of well-being, strength and energy, and decreased fatigue and sleepiness.

Persons with Klinefelter's syndrome have a low or easy threshold for developing behavior disabilities. The diversity of the symptoms manifested in affected individuals precludes the establishment of a specific psychiatric diagnosis to accompany the 47, XXY syndrome. Major symptoms of behavioral disability of the type found in XXY men in psychiatric and penal institutions have shown the same nosological diversity as have major symptoms of XY men in the same institutions, with no single diagnosis predominating. As culled from many sources, the disabilities include: schizophrenia, paranoia, suicidism, obsessional anxiety, phobia, pseudologia fantastica, transexualism, depression, alcoholism, criminal delinquency, sex offending, epilepsy, gross mental deficiency, and others. The prevalence of the syndrome in institutions for either gross mental deficiency or law-breaking behavior is higher than in the population at large. The exact figures for institutionalization vary with national and regional policies and facilities.

It seems perfectly feasible that the extra X chromosome in the nucleus of every cell in the brain somehow or another makes the organism more vulnerable to the risk of developing behavioral disabilities in a 47, XXY male as compared to a 46, XY male. Counseling means prevention, not just diagnosis or treatment in psychological medicine. A psychodynamic appraisal and counseling of the family may prevent conflicts before they exert their deleterious effects upon the patient.

It is possible that the years of puberty and adolescence are years of special, though not exclusive, risk for the development of behavioral disability. This is especially true for those XXY boys whose bodies virilize poorly, or whose sexual apathy makes them feel socially outcast. The decisive factor may not be inadequate adolescent development, per se, but the way in which other people react to it, and the pressure they may bring to bear on the boy. Sex, somatic stigmatization, and independence are three fundamental sources of conflict which the counselor should be prepared to deal with at this time.

CASE ILLUSTRATION

This patient's history at The Johns Hopkins Hospital began at the age of 19 when he was admitted to the psychiatric service upon the recommendation of his family physician. At this time, the presenting complaints were nervousness, shaking, and "butterflies in the stomach" whenever he left home or met someone new. These symptoms had been exacerbated 2 weeks prior to admission, to the point where the patient was unable to function adequately at his job (see biographical statement on p. 175).

A psychiatric diagnosis of "pseudoneurotic schizophrenia" was made. A medical student recommended a buccal smear, which proved to be chromatin positive. The ensuing full chromosome count disclosed a mosaic karyotype, 47,XXY/46,XY. After the diagnosis of Klinefelter's syndrome had been confirmed in the adult genetics clinic of The Johns Hopkins Hospital, the patient was referred for psychohormonal evaluation and counseling.

In an unsuccessful attempt to stimulate the growth of the patient's underdeveloped testes at age 7, the family physician had injected hormones of unspecified type. Pubertal development was spontaneous in onset at 15 years of age. Sexual and axillary hair were adequate. The penis remained small, and likewise the testes. There was mild gynecomastia.

Many aspects of the patient's behavorial history exemplify the inadequate personality type commonly found in men with the XXY syndrome. As a child, he tired easily from strenuous activity, and because he could not perform on a par with his peers, he participated in athletics infrequently. During his school years he preferred solitary activities such as reading, yet did enjoy camping and handicrafts as a Boy Scout.

At age 19, the Wechsler Adult Intelligence Test showed the full IQ to be 111 (Verbal IQ 106; Performance IQ 116).

Since his first and only psychiatric admission 11 years ago, at his own request, the patient has been maintained in monthly follow-up counseling by members of the psychohormonal research unit. In addition, he has been maintained on androgen therapy, testosterone enanthate 1.5 cc (300 mg) every 2 weeks, for the past 5 years. The initial effect was to give a mild, but satisfactory increase in somatic virilization, and a corresponding increase in masculine erotic interest and imagery, and in the frequency of erection and ejaculation. Sexual activity remained limited to masturbation and was not frequent. After 2 years, there was a change in sexual activity as the patient took up occasional dating with a woman from his place of work. She was sexually unsatisfied in her marriage. As a sequel to an automobile accident, her face had been scarred. The patient said that he enjoyed protecting, comforting, and looking after her. They had engaged in necking and petting, and had twice tried coitus, unsuccessfully, owing to premature ejaculation. This woman was almost twice his own age. This gerontophiliac tendency is always evident, if he feels any degree of romantic attraction toward a woman. There is no history of romantic attraction toward males.

Since his hospitalization, the patient has been receiving antianxiety medication, either Valium (diazepam) or Serax (oxazepam) in addition to androgen. His main problem can be characterized as a phobia of unfamiliar places, persons, and especially of driving in an automobile anywhere except the short distance to work. He has personally initiated many attempts to circumvent this phobia. The attempt generates anxiety culminating in an anxiety attack complete with dyspnea, tachycardia, trembling, flushing, and sweating. In the patient's own words, "It sometimes gets so bad my throat tightens up and I feel like I'll choke to death." He is able to get some relief by talking about upcoming threats to his equilibrium, such as what will happen to him if his parents leave the house to go on vacation, though even the talk is likely to precipitate sweating, hand tremor, and vocal tremor. He jokes sometimes about the predicament he is in, but has not been able to achieve the freedom from symptoms he would like.

Six months ago, aged nearly 30, the patient wrote the following brief biographical document as a sequel to a counseling session:

> In regards to our last conversation about doing a chromosome count at birth, I still have some pros and cons, since giving the time to think about it. Yes, I must agree it should be done. Tracing my own life back as far as I can remember, if this hidden factor would have been known perhaps 29 years ago, it's possible I would not be in the predicament that I am in now.
>
> My mother will verify that the first seven years of my life, I was rather sickly and extremely thin. You wouldn't know it now, though, would you? At age 7, I was operated on for a hernia. I don't know the particular reason for this. . . . I believe it was thought to be the cause of my having an upset stomach every morning. It worked for a while . . . but my stomach still makes a lot of acid.
>
> Back to my memory—at age 8, we moved to where I still live. These were of course pretty good years. My school work was always average, nothing exceptional. As you may find with some boys, not all of them though, if a subject does not interest them, there is no way they are going to learn it. So I remember quite a few low grades, even

then. Around this time, I remember my first contact with competitive sports, baseball, football, and any running sport. I really couldn't keep up with the other boys. I even joined a little league, believe it or not, on the advice of a doctor to get exercise. . . . I played two games and quit. Now I know some people are good at one thing and some are good at others, but when you don't understand how someone your own age (as I remember the rest of the team) could hit a ball so far, or run so fast, it brought to my mind: What's the matter with me? I believe it may have even then reduced me to tears. I decided for myself that I couldn't take the ribbing so I quit. . . . Again in school were games that were organized without any supervision. To be not wanted as a member of a team because you were not good enough, or not fast enough, or whatever, leaves a deep scar. So from third grade to the eighth grade I avoided any recess activities. My time was spent either walking through the school yard or as a cleaner. It may sound wierd, but this was a privilege. It meant you could stay inside. You could talk, you could read, or help the teachers with any little problems which made you feel good inside, any way.

At age 11, I joined the Boy Scouts. This was somewhat more rigorous, but it really had its benefits. There are things I learned in there that I still use today. I went camping. I loved the woods. I liked being out of doors. I still had no interest in girls, though, even though some of my friends did talk to them or even play with them (games that is).

At age 13 I entered high school in September. November that year I turned 14. . . . The school I attended, you won't believe it, did not have a physical education course. This was the main reason I wanted to go there. Another problem that developed in Scouts was that when you get a bunch of boys together, especially in a scout camp, nothing is private, believe me. And on shower day it all hangs out. Yes, I was embarrassed by kids saying I looked like a girl because of my chest development and my, shall we say, undersized penis. So by attending a school that was so far out in the boondocks, they could hardly supply water for regular toilet purposes. They sure as hell wouldn't be able to accommodate public showers. Again I avoided the embarrassment and the athletic letdown. . . . On the subject of girls again, I had very little contact, although I did talk to them, and did on occasion discuss their assets with the other boys. This is how 95% of the boys learn sex education. I guess we all had our fantasies, and there were a few girls that we picked out that we would really like to have sex with. Again these were fantasies. To the best of my knowledge none of these guys made, shall we say, made our dreams come true. I was either too shy or, from previous embarrassments I avoided most contacts with girls. I didn't go to my junior or senior proms. I don't even remember what excuses I used, but I did receive a great deal of ribbing about not being able to get a girl (at age 16 and no girl friend, that's pretty bad, regardless of what you or any doctors may preach). My friends around here weren't of much help, either, even though they were dating and bragging about their accomplishments. A few feels and some heavy petting—I was still in the woods, and we more or less drifted apart. . . .

Around this time another problem developed. Acne. After thousands of washings and an assortment of creams, jellies, etc., the doctor recommended hormone shots to speed up the puberty development. And it did. It cured my acne, and the shots were discontinued.

At age 16, I joined the fire house. I was in my glory now. I was probably the youngest fireman around, and probably the weakest, too. You really don't know how heavy 50 feet of old republic hose is until you try to pick it up over your head. . . . I enjoyed the friendship of the men and again the glory, and since these guys were mature, I took no ribbing about my physical appearance.

At age 17, I believe, I started on a mild tranquilizer, under doctor's care, again for nerves. Again the upset stomach and shakiness. . . ." [Not completed. He took ambulance training. A traumatic rescue experience precipitated the breakdown that required his psychiatric hospitalization.]

The foregoing biographical statement clearly conveys what it means personally to be growing up odd. Knowledge of the etiology of his oddity would not have lessened the primary problems, but it would have alerted teachers and family to the role they might have played in reducing an overlay of secondary problems by expecting too much conformity to the stereotype of the all-American boy.

At the present time, the patient has a commonsense knowledge of the facts of his own case. There is nothing that he can learn behind the scenes regarding his diagnosis that will frighten him—nothing from reading or television regarding 47,XXY—and nothing that will catch him unprepared. Diagnostic knowledge has helped him, and his family too, to plan his medical and psychologic care more rationally, by knowing what probabilities and expectancies they should plan for. His progress has been slow, but it has not been negative, and the prognosis, though limited, at least is not worsened by reason of a false diagnosis.

47,XYY Syndrome

SIGNS AND SYMPTOMS

There is no characteristic that is uniformly present in patients with 47,XYY chromosome constitution other than the fact that they do have an extra Y chromosome. Tall stature is, however, a very common somatic sign among these individuals. Clinically, they may have neurologic disturbance. Some have various types of skeletal abnormality and post-pubertal facial acne. Dermatoglyphically, there is a higher frequency of arches on the finger tip, a somewhat lower total finger ridge count than in 46,XY males, and a hypothenar pattern on the sole. There is increased frequency of both high and low androgen levels. Other frequently found physical characteristics include: low birth weight, grossly abnormal brain waves as measured by electroencephalogram, hyperactivity or other disturbances in locomotor activity, impaired testicular cells (sterility or reduced fertility), skin disorders, and dental abnormalities.

Incidence studies of the frequency of the 47,XYY karyotype in morphologic males at birth were laboriously slow and expensive until the discovery in 1970 of the flourescent staining technique for rapid screening of Y chromosomes. Today, progress is further hindered in the United States by the aftermath of misguided claims that karyotyping of infants would lead to their being branded guilty of criminality by karyotype, prior to their being old enough to commit a crime. At the present time, therefore, the frequency incidence of XYY in the newborn is uncertain. Different studies have produced an estimated incidence ratio of 1:975 live births, the range varying from 0:2000 to 1:250.

BEHAVIORAL CHARACTERISTICS

Behavioral disabilities in the case of the XYY karyotype became unjustifiably stereotyped because of the type of institution in which the karyotype first became easy to find. With the title of the first report in 1965 by Jacobs and coworkers, "Aggressive Behaviour, Mental Subnormality and the XYY Male," XYY became the aggressive stereotype. The media took up the stereotype. Almost overnight the supernumerary Y chromosome became, alas, the crime chromosome. Prevalence studies were, for the next few years, directed towards tall males in prisons or institutions for the criminally insane. Today, in consequence, prevalence statistics are informative only with respect to XYY men who have gotten into trouble with the law. Information about those who do not tangle with the law is either negligible or anecdotal, and not statistically systematic. Nonetheless, it is of significant importance to know that some quiet-living XYY men have been discovered, for example by Noel and Revin (1974) in France.

Investigators have focused so much attention on aggression and criminality in the XYY syndrome that other behavioral traits were overlooked. The most noteworthy oversight, initially, was with respect to sexual behavior. In addition to consensual homosexuality or bisexuality, the incidence of socially uncondoned sexual behavior appears to be elevated. Reports of such behavior include bisexual child incest, pedophilia, voyeurism, exhibitionism, transvestism, indecent assault, sadomasochism, and in one instance, sex murder.

Tabulating behavioral data from 31 published cases, plus 4 studied in detail at The Johns Hopkins Hospital, Money and coworkers in 1970 listed various forms of behavior that may prove to be pathognomonic, albeit not universally distributed in the XYY syndrome. The list is: difficult child; problems in school; excessive daydreaming; loner; drifter; unrealistic future expectations; impulsiveness; sudden violence and aggression; imprisonment; homosexual plus heterosexual tendencies; paraphilias. The frequency of low IQ in the XYY male is an unknown. Nonetheless, it is known that average and high IQ's are compatible with the XYY chromosomal complement.

If one searches for a common denominator of all the traits or disabilities of behavior, it may well be an impairment of the brain's function of inhibition at the interface where image is translated into action. In more familiar terms, one might say that XYY boys and men are highly impulsive, flighty in attention span, and not good at self-regulation of behavior. In ordinary behavioral development, one expects impulsive, poorly self-regulated behavior to be in varying degree characteristic of the years of infancy and immaturity. Such immaturity seems to be greatly prolonged in XYY individuals, so that in the years of young adulthood, for example, they are still behaving as juveniles or young adolescents. There is some evidence to suggest that they do eventually catch up in behavioral maturation, provided they survive the vicissitudes of the years of prolonged lagging behind.

COUNSELING

When a 47,XYY child, adolescent, or adult first enters our clinic with a history of antisocial behavior, he has long been the victim of a principle, both overt and covert, in the folk philosophy of our times, namely, that if he really tried to he could control his behavior voluntarily. In like manner, the folk philosophy spelled out in some instances by professionals may have victimized parents by telling them that they must have done, or must still be doing something wrong to produce their son's abnormal behavior. Implied guilt of this type has a noxious and often adverse effect on the subsequent behavior of both the patient and his family. The situation is as traumatic as if a patient with epilepsy were led to believe that he and his family are behaviorally responsible for his seizures.

It is easier for XYY boys and men to benefit from counseling, if they know that they are the fortuitous victims of a handicap, and not simply the behavioral product of a faulty upbringing, or of self-induced failure. One of the surest ways to gain their trust and an eventual improvement in self-regulation of behavior is by way of communicating one's understanding that they are subject to a degree of behavioral impulsiveness unfamiliar to the ordinary person. Thus, for the family and community of an XYY male to learn that he has a supernumerary Y chromosome may completely change their concept of the cause of his impulsive and socially stigmatized behavior. Self-blame can be lifted. The self-righteous morality of punishment as a means of training and reform can be replaced by a new morality of incentive and reward training.

There is some observational evidence of a preliminary nature to suggest that an XYY child has particular difficulty negotiating the ordinary demands of socialization, and that the demands on the parents of such a child for excellence and expertise in child rearing are greater than those required by their other children. The XYY's risk for developing behavioral disability related to impulsiveness in its varying manifestations can be, to some degree, ameliorated by a benign environment of rearing, instead of aggravated by a socially malignant environment. Even in a benign environment, the parents and other responsible adults may need to be exceptionally well-trained and counseled in child rearing. Otherwise they may be rendered behaviorally incompetent and disabled themselves by the exceptional and taxing demands of the task of rearing an XYY boy.

There are some XYY men with disabling antisocial behavior of an impulsive and sexual type whose rehabilitation is helped by a course of antiandrogen medication, and with counseling. Of the two best-tested antiandrogens, cyproterone acetate and medroxyprogesterone acetate, only the latter has been cleared for use in the United States. Medroxyprogesterone acetate has been found to have an effect on sexual behavior in both the 47,XYY and 46,XY genotypes. This effect can be rated as beneficial when sexual behavior is of a paraphiliac type which is socially not tolerated, but severely punished. The effect is manifested not only as a diminution or suppression of erection and ejaculation, along with suppression of testicular androgen, but also as a lessening of the frequency and compulsiveness of erotic imagery. All of these changes are reversible upon withdrawal of treatment. In some instances, the effect is not only reversible but brings with it a change of imagery from a paraphiliac and socially stigmatized type to a socially acceptable type. Such a degree of change represents, so to speak, a psychic realignment, which probably cannot take place without the concurrent effect of counseling.

CASE ILLUSTRATION

The patient, now 24, was first brought to the psychohormonal research unit at age 15 for interviewing and psychological testing, 1 year after he had been identified as having a chromosomal constitution of XYY. The boy was first referred to his school counselor at age 6 as a newly admitted student. His mother explained that "he had violent temper fits and at times would wreck his toys and belongings." He was enuretic until age 8 or 9 and was described as slow and a dreamer. His daydreams, according to his mother, were quite real to him. Although the boy was subject to violent fits of temper at times, he was not a constant bullying, aggressive person.

At the time of the school report, his thinking showed signs of perseveration. His perception of his environment was described as unusual and, at times, bordering on the bizarre. The report indicated that the boy hallucinated and it characterized him as being uncertain of himself when dealing with others. During his early months as a first grader, the boy's academic work was very poor. He was known to behave peculiarly at times, as the report observed,

> pulling a sweater over his head and putting his head down. He hears voices at times, seems confused and in a daze. His attention span is extremely short, and his social relationships are few. He has only one good friend, and has been known, at times, to hit other children with no apparent reason.

The subsequent history of this boy has been one of steady improvement, even with regard to his EEG, which was abnormal at age 10½ years, showing a typical seizure spike. His IQ at this age was in the dull–normal range, as it had been when first tested at age 6. But at age 15, it was normal, and his nonverbal IQ was 111, putting it into the bright–normal range. Based on these several criteria, one can infer that the boy is making progress and has tended to grow out of his difficulties.

Between ages 10 and 15, the boy changed remarkably. This change was owing in part to his having been enrolled in a special school for the so-called brain-damaged, where some of the pressure of an ordinary schoolroom orientation toward achievement was taken off him. Equally important, however, was the effort put forth by his parents. Before the correct diagnosis was made of his chromosomal abnormality, his parents were often covertly blamed for his lack of self-control and other behavioral difficulties. They were indirectly accused of shirking their responsibility as parents in his upbringing. Once he was diagnosed, they felt relieved that his difficulties had not been of their doing, and that they could now begin working to attempt to correct his problem. Here one sees an excellent example of the way in which society can, literally, prevent therapeutic action from taking place because blame for someone's condition is misplaced.

Episodically, the patient was liable to regress and manifest peculiar behavior. At age 12 a report came from his teacher that he appears to be distracted for various periods of time throughout the day, talking and apparently listening to someone who is not there. He moves his lips, nods his head, raises his eyebrows, and chuckles or laughs. I have seen signs that make me believe he is masturbating in his cubicle in the classroom.

At age 15, he was returned to a regular classroom. Mistakenly, he was placed in a class of rough children who were not highly achieved. Apparently, during that period of time, the teachers were forced to reprimand loudly all of the students in that class. The boy had been assigned to this class because of his own underachievement, as well as his prior difficult behavior. As it turned out, he overreacted and took personally the teachers' reprimanding of the entire class. In consequence, he had difficulty sleeping at night, and his behavior began to deteriorate.

The two school reports suggest that abrupt change from a familiar environment to a strange one was for him a very special source of stress, almost a trauma, under which his behavior deteriorated.

He grew up to share common tendencies of XYY adults to be daydreamers and loners, to relate as they sit and talk, in a friendly and pleasant, though transient way, and to minimize continuity and carry-through in relationships. He planned his activities on an isolationist basis, so that one could not quite predict what might develop in the future.

Presently, the patient is progressing surprisingly well, despite the limitation of being socially a loner. He recalled no more than one or two tantrum-like outbursts in the years between ages 18 and 24. The most recent one was so upsetting to his parents that they requested a special appointment.

Upon graduation from a special school for slow learners, he found employment at a large factory where he earns a self-supporting salary. His recreations include target shooting with a .22 rifle, and bowling once a week. He has not, as yet, begun dating and has not experienced any sexual activity other than masturbation. He follows his parents in being devoutly religious and a regular church goer. He reads and follows the Holy Scriptures. Through his church group, he participates in dinner gatherings, softball games, and youth group trips to the ocean. He enjoys participating in all of these activities.

Without knowledge of this patient's chromosomal aberration, it is highly probable that professional planning on his behalf would have progressed entirely differently. Until the chromosomes were counted, his behavior disorder was attributed exclusively to a psychogenic etiology, with its hidden implication of parental responsibility. It should not, of course, require a chromosome count to justify the removal of covert blame from parents, but the fact of the matter is that professional people today seem to need tangible evidence of a "physical cause" before they can properly distribute the etiological components of a disorder. The issue is not one of organic versus psychogenic, for the development of the parent–child relationship is always important, regardless of the organic substrate. Knowledge of the boy's chromosomal status in this case took some of the heat off the parents, allowing them and professionals to work together in mutual understanding of what they had to cope with. The outcome, in term's of the boy's behavioral progress, was enhanced. Professional time, effort, and expense were reduced. Follow-up counseling eventually could be scheduled on a self-demand basis. It continues that way, and the demand is very infrequent.

Summary

Applied behavioral genetics is a new branch of psychology, knowledge of which facilitates the psychotherapeutic process for patients diagnosed as having one of three cytogenetic syndromes: 45,X (Turner's); 47,XXY (Klinefelter's); and the 47,XYY syndrome.

Behaviorally, Turner's syndrome is characterized by space–form (praxic) disability, inertia of emotional arousal, feminine gender identity, and maternal interests. Two pathognomonic signs of the syndrome are short stature and lack of functioning ovaries. The task of the counselor in dealing effectively with patients with Turner's syndrome includes explaining the diagnosis to the patient, supporting her through difficult decisions, and aiding her in coping with the stigmata of the syndrome.

Presence of a supernumerary X or Y chromosome increases the risk that an individual will develop behavioral disability. Such disability in individuals with 47,XXY (Klinefelter's) syndrome is often characterized by impairment, deficiency, or inhibition of doing, while persons with the 47,XYY syndrome develop disability characterized by overdoing something, on an impulsive basis, with poor planning regarding long-term outcome. In revealing the chromosomal anomaly as the putative source of the patient's behavioral difficulties, the counselor facilitates removal of self-blame from the patient and/or family. In XYY men, if there are sexual problems with the law, the patient may benefit from a term of antiandrogen treatment. Conversely, sexual inadequacy in XXY men may be helped with testosterone therapy.

In all three syndromes the task of the counselor in dealing with a patient includes explaining the diagnosis in terms that are understandable and nontraumatizing, formulating personally acceptable ways of coping with the stigmata of the syndrome, and elucidating alternatives when personal decisions must be negotiated.

References

Alexander, D. & Money, J. Turner's syndrome and Gerstmann's syndrome: Neuropsychologic comparisons. *Neuropsychologia*, 1966, *4*, 265–273.
Bird, B. *Talking with patients.* 2nd ed. Philadelphia: Lippincott, 1973.
Blocker, D. *Developmental counseling.* New York: Ronald Press, 1966.
Gardner, L. I. (ed.). *Endocrine and genetic diseases of childhood and adolescence.* 2nd ed. Philadelphia: Saunders, 1975.
Hambert, G. *Males with positive sex chromatin: An epidemiologic investigation followed by psychiatric study of seventy-five cases.* Göteborg: Elanders Boktryckeri Aktiebolag, 1966.
Jacobs, P., Brunton, M., Melville, M., Brittain, R. & McClemont, W. Aggressive behaviour, mental sub-normality and the XYY male. *Nature*, 1965, *208*, 1351–1352.
Lindsten, J. *The nature and origin of X chromosome aberrations in Turner's syndrome.* Stockholm: Almquist and Wiksell, 1963.
Money, J. *Sex errors of the body: Dilemmas, education and counseling.* Baltimore: Johns Hopkins Press, 1968.
Money, J. Human behavior cytogenetics: Review of psychopathology in three syndromes, 47,XXY; 47,XYY; and 45,X. *Journal of Sex Research*, 1975, *11*: 181–200.
Money, J., Annecillo, C., Van Orman, B. & Borgaonkar, D. S. Cytogenetics, hormones and behavior disability: Comparison of XYY and XXY syndromes. *Clinical Genetics*, 1974, *6*, 370–382.
Money, J. & Ehrhardt, A. A. *Man and woman, boy and girl: The differentiation and dimorphism of gender identity from conception to maturity.* Baltimore: Johns Hopkins Press, 1972.
Money, J., Gaskin, R. and Hull, H. Impulse, aggression and sexuality in the XYY syndrome. *St. John's Law Review*, 1970, *44*, 220–235.
Money, J. & Mittenthal, S. Lack of personality pathology in Turner's syndrome: Relation to cytogenetics, hormones and physique. *Behavior Genetics*, 1970, *1*, 43–56.
Murken, J. The XYY Syndrome and Klinefelter's Syndrome. Vol. 2 of *Topics in Human Genetics.* (P. E. Becker, W. Lenz, F. Vogel, G. G. Wendt, eds.), Stuttgart, Germany: Georg Thieme, 1973.
Nielsen, J. *Klinefelter's syndrome and the XYY syndrome: A genetical endocrinological and psychiatric-psychological study of 33 hypogonadal male patients and 2 patients with karyotype 47, XYY.* Copenhagen, Denmark: Munksgaard, 1969.
Noel, B. & Revil, D. Some personality perspectives of XYY individuals taken from the general population. *Journal of Sex Research*, 1974, *10*, 219–225.
Watson, M. A. & Money, J. Behavior cytogenetics and Turner's syndrome: A new principle in counseling and psychotherapy. *American Journal of Psychotherapy*, 1975, *29*, 166–177.
Witkin, H. A., Mednick, S. A., Schulsinger, F., Bakkerstrom, E., Christiansen, K. O., Goodenough, D. R., Hirschhorn, K., Lundsteen, C., Owen, D. R., Philip, J., Rubin, D. B. & Stocking, M. Criminality in XYY and XXY men. *Science*, 1976, *193*, 547–555.

Psychological Issues in Sickle Cell Counseling

11

Verle E. Headings

Since serious activity in sickle cell counseling dates only to about 1971, any perspective on this topic is yet in its infancy. The experience of the intervening years has, however, created the material from which rigorously designed investigations may emerge. Throughout this discussion, salient issues encountered by genetic counselors will be discussed and a particular emphasis will be given to the psychological aspects of counseling for sickle cell pertinent to different life stages. Promising research directions will be outlined at points where these are germane.

Self Image and Sickle Cell

Sickle cell, like any chronic disorder, exerts a defining effect on the person's self-image. The effects of the disorder are usefully separated into those of a purely biological character, those found in social discourse and public image of sickle cell, those associated with a given life stage, and the effects of interaction with a person's ethnic minority status.

To more fully appreciate the ramifications of a sickle cell-related self-image for the health of the individual, the following definitions of health will be employed. "Health is defined broadly as harmony, balance, dynamic equilibrium both between organism and environment and among the organism's constituent parts, a condition that is possible only if the organism has the capacity to adapt to constantly changing circumstances [Mischel, 1977]." Also, "for most people, in fact, health does not mean

185

GENETIC COUNSELING
Psychological Dimensions

so much the absence of disease as the ability to conduct life according to personal choices and social conventions [Dubos, 1977]." Hopefully, it will become apparent that the various types of impact of sickle cell on one's self-image do indeed distort the usual equilibrium between individuals and their environment. Later, I will examine in detail a genetic counseling model designed to safeguard the personal choices and adaptability of individuals with sickle cell trait or disease.

Sickle cell trait exerts no substantial biological impairment on the person and hence it exerts no biological impact on self-image. The biological effects of sickle cell disease, on the other hand, are of a waxing and waning nature, allowing the individual to pursue activities that must then be curtailed during times of sickling crises. This effectively cuts into the person's ability to hold certain types of employment or to engage in physically demanding ventures. In the school age child, the young adult, or in the parent, this repeated experience may burden the individual with images of personal incompetence. For example, young people on occasion have chosen not to acquire a college education because of low self expectations. Low expectations too frequently are reinforced by family, health care providers, and educational counselors. An appropriate research design should both quantify the person's self-image of incompetence and the sources of such an image.

The knowledge that one's life span is frequently shortened by sickle cell disease may place limits on the individual's expectations, producing a fatalism and an unreadiness to live to his or her full potential.

The public images and social discourse about sickle cell have undoubtable impact on the self-image of individuals with either the trait or the disease. All inherited conditions with the potential for physical disability tend to carry a stigma for the family. For some uninformed individuals, this stigma has been associated, on occasion, with a belief that sickle cell is contagious. To carry this further, some health professionals draw an analogy between the risk of sickle cell disease among children of carrier parents and the risk of contagious disease. The public image of "defectiveness" in the individual's biology, necessitating publicly financed programs to prevent its recurrence, unwittingly may convince the individual with sickle cell trait or disease that society is opposed to the type of individual represented. At times, fund raising campaigns for the treatment of and research on sickle cell disease portray the undesirable features of this genetic "scourge," labeling it as a killer. This public discourse, in the name of benevolence, is clearly insensitive to the self-image of persons with either trait or disease. The relatively high frequency of sickle cell trait in some populations invites a belief, on the part of some, that such populations are marked and constitute groups of less adequate ancestry than other populations.

Major research on stigmatization is needed in order to quantify the extent to which the individual with trait or disease perceives these effects in the various social contexts. Likewise, the extent to which individuals in those contexts actually project negative attitudes and behaviors toward persons with trait or disease should be documented.

The presence of sickle cell in youths and in potential parents interacts significantly with one's images of sexual and parenting competence. At a life stage when there is relatively more uncertainty in these matters, the revelation by a health professional that the trait, or disease is present makes the grasp on certainty even more tenuous. This can be inadvertently exacerbated by the counselor who employs imagery that is loaded for the client. For example, to speak about sickle cell as a "condition of the blood" is very parallel to the "bad blood" imagery many lay persons employ for undesirable hereditary traits. Furthermore when the counselor links a discussion of a recurrence risk with reproduction, the client may conclude erroneously that sexual or reproductive incompetence is implied.

For many individuals, ethnic status becomes a component of their self-image. If one puts together minority ethnic status, and a long history of socioeconomic disadvantage with a relatively high risk of sickle cell disease, some individuals conclude that either there is a cause–effect relationship between minority status and sickle cell, or else that members of ethnic majorities have fabricated such a relationship. In either case, the acceptability of a given ethnic identity is perceived as being under assault.

It has been postulated that sickle cell disease creates physical limitations which, in turn, may promote a negative body image. To the extent that racism creates conditions that promote negative body symbols, this may set up a faulty body imagery, which in turn hampers the ability to cope with the stresses of sickle cell disease (Phillips, 1973).

Misconceptions about Sickle Cell

A substantial element of counseling for sickle cell concerns misconceptions of fact and the accompanying emotional distress. A sampling of these misconceptions follows:

1. Sickle cell "trait" is a *trace* of sickle cell disease; it may worsen with time; and individuals do die from it. This confusion is unfortunately abetted by the choice of the term *trait* for the carrier state and is a problem for uninformed health professionals as well as for lay persons. The term trait is commonly used to refer to a genetic phenotype. Historically, its application to sickle cell was an exception, in which trait was reserved for the carrier state identifiable by cell sickling, but without a

clinical phenotype. The counselor might promote more clarity by using the terminology of S-carrier rather than sickle cell trait.

2. Sickle cell is contagious via sexual intercourse or other intimate physical contact. A 23-year-old man was presented to a genetics clinic with multiple physical complaints and firmly believed that he was symptomatic for sickle cell disease. He believed also that he had acquired sickle cell disease from his girl friend, who reportedly had sickle cell trait, by contact with menstrual blood during sexual intercourse. On testing, this man was proven to have sickle cell trait, a fact he refused to acknowledge. The conversation of this client generally reflected irrational content, particularly concerning fears about his health. The situation does illustrate the manner by which misconceptions can be linked one to another in order to rationalize a phobia or an untenable personal situation, such as lack of success in securing a job. In this instance one sees misconceptions of attributing inconsistent physical complaints to a feared diagnosis, acquiring sickle cell by contact with blood of someone with sickle cell (the bad blood imagery), and trait changes into disease.

3. Sickle cell is specifically related to skin pigmentation. This misconception is an extension of the commonly expressed belief that sickle cell disease is a "black disease." If not corrected, it reinforces long held negative interracial relationships by both white and black individuals. By generalization, this misconception may serve to stigmatize an ethnic minority status. On the other hand, it may serve to promote the view that sickle cell is a fiction created by a white power structure in order to place blacks in a relatively subordinate position.

4. Sickle cell trait in only one parent poses a risk of sickle cell disease among offspring. This usually reflects a lack of understanding of how genes are related to clinical diseases. However, when a client expresses this belief to the counselor, the latter ought to be aware that the client may be exposing his or her most extreme fears in order to receive reassurance that they are groundless.

5. Sickle cell disease allows no hope for a fulfilling life. This misconception is frequently fostered by mass media portrayals of this condition or by contact with persons who have sickle cell disease and whose medical care was less than optimal.

Apprehensions about Restrictions on Social Opportunity

When individuals with sickle cell disease have lost their jobs, not infrequently, the employers have justified their action with arguments that a hazard to health existed or that the employee lacked sufficient skills.

In the face of a good employment record, the individual with sickle cell disease is faced with an elusive form of discrimination which is frequently difficult to challenge successfully. Ill-informed employers do not appreciate the possibilities for tailoring work situations to the individual's physical requirements or, on the other hand, may be following a stereotyped belief that one should stay clear of individuals with bad blood. In either case, the effect is a socially instigated restriction on personal choices based on beliefs concerning an inherited disease. There can be no doubt that this situation increases the psychological burden accompanying sickle cell; this is the converse of health as defined by Dubos (1977) earlier in this chapter.

Experiences of individuals with sickle cell trait have included being restricted on athletic activity at higher altitudes, being refused employment as airline stewardesses, increased life insurance rates, and being refused entrance into military service. Beyond the practical effects on such individuals, the not-so hidden message of such experiences is that there is an institutionalized perception that sickle cell trait represents defectiveness (Murray, 1976).

Although apprehension about the marriageability of individuals with sickle cell trait has not been adequately examined, there is reason to suspect that it is of substantial magnitude, given the types of misconceptions presented by individuals who seek counseling for sickle cell trait. For example, in the social context of a village in Greece, where marriages are arranged by the family and, where extensive testing and counseling were carried out, individuals with sickle cell trait found themselves shunned as marriage partners (Stamatoyannopoulos, 1974).

Given the fact of adverse responses by many institutions and individuals to persons with sickle cell trait, the latter frequently feel constrained to hide their sickle cell status. The life-long risk that such information may inadvertently get into the wrong hands poses a potential psychological burden.

Iatrogenic Complications of Testing and Counseling

The process of informing an individual that he or she has sickle cell trait introduces the risk of an adverse experience, already discussed in the sections on self-image and social restrictions, without providing any direct health benefit to the individual. These potential complications must be a central feature of the counseling experience if they are not to obscure the potential benefits.

The potential benefits seem to rest entirely on the premise that informed decision making by prospective parents about the prevention of diseases will improve the future health of individuals and the well-being of families. This does not translate into no risk-taking in every high risk recurrence situation. Rather, it may prepare parents to adapt to and accept, in a mature way, the outcome of their conscious risk-taking.

A highly directive counselor will tend to hold to the view that the prevention of the birth of a child with sickle cell disease is the paramount goal of counseling. It appears that pediatricians and internists tend toward more directiveness in this situation than do individuals in the counseling professions (Headings, 1976). In the view of this writer, directive counseling toward the goal of prevention represents an iatrogenic consequence of testing in that it subordinates the individual's decision making, choices, and self-determination to that of professional goals.

Another iatrogenic consequence of testing and counseling can be an inadvertent exposure of nonpaternity. In other words, the putative biological father's hemoglobin phenotype is found to be incompatible with that of his child's. It has been estimated that nonpaternity in some segments of the United States population may range as high as 15%. The risk of imposing severe emotional trauma on the spouse or child can be minimized by the perceptive counselor in several ways:

1. The testing of parents should be discouraged in circumstances where there is no occasion for informed decision making about the recurrence of sickle cell disease.

   A 19-year-old college student was tested in a routine screening program offered to all entering students at a university. She was found to have sickle cell trait. During the follow-up counseling she expressed the intention of encouraging both of her parents to be tested. The counselor pointed out that since they were past child bearing age there was no benefit to be gained by such information except possibly to satisfy their curiosity.

2. In circumstances where both young parents are seeking testing, the counselor can mention the sources of discrepancy between parent and offspring phenotypes in explaining the potential outcomes of testing. This, at least, provides an informed basis for either parent to decide against testing if either fears the disclosure of socially disruptive information.

Screening programs in elementary schools or those which encourage screening for the entire family are likely to reveal situations in which both parents have an AA hemoglobin phenotype, as do each of their children, except one who has an AS phenotype. They may not have had prior information about the inheritance of sickle cell and may request an appointment with the genetic counselor. In such a circumstance some counselors elect to interpret the child's S gene as an instance of new mutation. Others, however, see this as jeopardizing the counselor's credibility as well as denying to the individual the responsibility for making their own, albeit difficult decisions. An alternative approach in such situations is for the counselor to communicate first with the mother apprising her of the discordant test results and its possible origins. If she has reason to believe that her child was fathered by another man, she can be encouraged to make a decision on how she wishes to deal with the dilemma. As we shall see later this is consistent with the counselor's role of functioning only as consultant and encouraging responsible decision making by the client.

A similar, but less complex situation might arise in newborn screening programs for sickle cell disease. Whenever an infant is identified as having sickle cell disease it is recommended that both parents be tested to confirm the recurrence risk for this specific mating pair. A sensitive counselor may, however, first interpret the expected and occasional discordant test results to the mother before the parents are tested. If she senses a risk of disclosing nonpaternity she can exercize her choice to avoid this possibility.

Psychological Effects of Sickle Cell Related to Stage of Life

A stage-of-life orientation to counseling for sickle cell has been notably missing in most literature in this area. Such an orientation has also been poorly developed in sickle cell screening services. Some services have produced ill-advised ventures, such as screening children in elementary schools and public appealing for entire families to be tested. Testing and counseling services must be inseparably linked, with a common objective of providing a specific health related benefit to the individual tested or the potential offspring. The specifics of the objective differ according to the life stage of the individual, and indeed at some stages the objective is not applicable.

In the postreproductive stage, the occasions for testing are indeed few in number. Individuals with clinically significant hemoglobinopathies are rarely initially ascertained at this age, and test information no longer contributes to decision making about the prevention of hemoglobinopathies in offspring. As indicated earlier, there is a substantial risk that testing at this stage will identify nonpaternity.

Finding the sickle cell trait during the adolescent and young adult stages of life can readily destabilize or stress those developmental needs of high priority during these stages. Thus, a concern to prove one's manhood or womanhood, an adequacy of sexual performance, and an ability to freely choose one's activities, may appear, to the individual, to be placed in jeopardy by this condition which "affects the blood." Ignorance, coupled with misconceptions, promotes anxiety, from which the individuals will develop their own rationale.

A young husband and wife without children learned that they were both carriers for sickle cell. After the initial phases of counseling, each developed a different level of apprehension about the one-in-four risk of occurrence of sickle cell disease. The wife would not consider taking such a risk whereas the husband wanted to proceed with a pregnancy. Research on the frequency and magnitude of marital friction and unsatisfactory sexual relationships arising from such situations is of high priority. The probability of such disagreements may indeed be higher for a condition such as sickle cell disease, where the morbidity is variable and discontinuous and where the disease is accompanied by a relatively less severe or universal social stigma than for conditions such as mental retardation and mental illness, which carry a relatively higher social stigma (Tringo, 1970).

An objective during the reproductive stage, both before and after marriage, is to provide options for dealing prospectively with the risk of occurrence of sickle cell disease among potential offspring. This concerns not only the prevention of the birth of a child with sickle cell disease, but also may allow potential parents to make an accommodation to their risk prior to an emotional investment in the child. It has been reported that parents who give birth to children with highly incapacitating genetic disorders experience feelings of guilt, a sense of interpersonal failure, and of being a doomed family (Agle, 1964; Langsley, 1961). This has not been adequately documented for parents of children with sickle cell disease. However, anecdotal information suggests that some degree of parental remorse about their act of producing a child with this condition does exist.

Newborn screening for sickle cell disease secures information of a discouraging nature precisely at a time when parents are celebrating a long awaited event. Furthermore, the diagnosis at this stage possesses an abstract quality since by parental inspection the infant appears to be in good health. Observations of parent–infant interaction during counseling sessions suggest that there is disbelief and denial of the possibility that the apparently healthy child carries a potential for much distress. Clearly, research of high priority is needed to define the spectrum of parental emotional experience in response to the birth of a child with sickle cell disease, both with and without counseling prior to the conception of such a child.

The identification of sickle cell trait in prereproductive children presents a situation where the risks usually surpass the potential benefits. The ascertainment of a child with sickle cell trait will occasionally identify a trait by trait mating involving parents who are still in their reproductive years. Against this must be placed the risk of exposing nonpaternity, the labeling of the child with a diagnosis which has no practical consequence at that life stage and the risk of introducing fear and possibly adversely affecting a child's self-image in its formative stages, especially if the child encounters adverse comments about sickle cell.

The identification of sickle cell disease in the fetus is an experimental procedure at this time, and hence, there has been insufficient opportunity to document possible psychological effects of such a diagnosis on the parents. Two concerns, raised in relation to the selective termination of pregnancy in other disorders, are also likely to pertain to sickle cell disease. The presence of guilt has been reported in a proportion of parents who choose abortion as a means for preventing inherited disorders. As the prenatal diagnosis of sickle cell disease becomes a realistic option, careful research will be required to enable counselors to identify those parents who may harbor unresolved personal moral dilemmas about abortion long after their decision is made. It is postulated that parents in such an unresolved situation may experience feelings of prolonged guilt after the abortion, which in turn could adversely affect the health of the parent, as defined by Mischel (1977) before. Resolution of any guilt feelings prior to proceeding with abortion may yield a better prognosis for the parent's health. Given the variability of clinical severity of this disorder as well as the diversity of opinion on abortion among the social peers of many parents, the risk of criticism about an abortion decision is not inconsequential. A parent who therefore can make an adaptation to an abortion decision prior to proceeding on it is less likely to be captive to guilt imputed by other persons.

A second concern pertains to parents who already have one child with a handicap and who contemplate prenatal diagnosis for subsequent pregnancies. Can the rejection of a midtrimester affected fetus be reconciled with a full investment in and identification with the first affected child? This question deserves particular attention for a condition like sickle cell disease with its substantial variability in clinical severity.

Content of Counseling

An examination of the content of sickle cell counseling needs to be prefaced with a statement about the relationships between the counselor and counselee (Headings, 1976). Most encounters between a health professional and a client find the former in a directive, decision-making role, whereas the latter often expects to be a relatively passive recipient of some corrective measure. In counseling for genetic disorders this situation should customarily be reversed. The counselor needs to affirm the counselee as an information gatherer, a decision maker, and as an implementer of decisions. To do so, the counselor needs to be a consultant and a facilitator.

The content of counseling for sickle cell will, of course, be tailored to the particular life stage of the individual and to the specific form of the sickling phenotype (AS, SS, SC, S-Thal, SG, SF). There is, however, a core of information that, in my experience, transcends life stage and phenotype and addresses the psychological issues identified. This content, outlined below, should be provided during the initial counseling session (Headings, 1975):

1. The structure and function of red blood cells and their hemoglobins.

2. The relationship between sickling hemoglobinopathies and red cell shape.

3. The consequences of red cell sickling *in vivo*—shortened red cell survival and small vessel obstruction—and the relationship of these to symptoms of sickle cell disease.

4. The inheritance of the hemoglobinopathy genes and the application of this knowledge for interpreting the individual's situation; that is, how he acquired them and the chances that he will transmit them.

5. The spectrum of complications associated with sickle cell disease.

6. Sickle cell trait is not considered a disease although higher than usual frequencies of urinary tract infection in pregnant women and hematuria are to be expected. Under rare circumstances of hypoxia intravascular sickling could occur and hence the client is encouraged to avoid such circumstances.

7. The variability in life span, the severity of complications of sickle cell disease, and the growing awareness that optimal general health care and tailoring of the individual's environment can reduce complications. Of particular recent importance are findings of significant frequencies of infant death from pneumonias and other infections (Powars, 1975). Diagnosis in the newborn infant is expected to lead to closer health monitoring, including the use of a recently developed vaccine for the pneumococcus, and to the prevention of deaths.

8. Geographic and racial distributions of sickle cell and comparative information about a sampling of other inherited disorders, such as phenylketonuria, cystic fibrosis, and Tay-Sachs disease. The laws of genetics are no respecter of persons—all groups are subject to inherited disorders.

9. The multiethnic distribution of sickle cell and its spread from various countries to the Americas.

10. The protective role of the sickle trait against falciparum malaria.

11. Alternatives for preventing the occurrence of sickle cell disease and conveying the importance of the realization that any actions on this represent a decision of the client.

12. Promising directions in research on prevention and treatment.

Many of these facts can be effectively reinforced with a desk top slide viewer. In the view of some health professionals these details may appear excessive in terms of time required (about 45 minutes) and the readiness of most clients to comprehend this information. Their value, however, must be judged, in part, on the way in which they deal with the psychological issues and the needs surrounding sickle cell.

Some of the psychological issues to which the above counseling content is addressed are as follows:

1. The facts presented may remove the mysteriousness, capriciousness, and erroneous hear-say elements of sickle cell, so that misconceptions can be corrected. For some individuals this helps to deal with the fear of the unknown. Even though it may be difficult to do so, that which is known and understood can be dealt with more realistically than that which is not known or understood.

2. There are options available for prevention, reducing morbidity, or optimizing the adaptation to a difficult situation.

3. Affirmation of the individual as significant irrespective of his hemoglobin phenotype.

4. Affirmation of the individual as decision maker about his or her situation.

5. The sickle gene, and very probably others, have beneficial as well as deleterious effects. It is erroneous to speak of "bad genes," "bad blood," and so on.

6. The client is not alone with his situation; the counselor is an empathetic and always available consultant, and medical investigators are actively seeking options for treatment and prevention. The clients can feel that they deserve to be taken into the counselor's confidence so that the former realize the counselor is a partner in finding ways to meaningful solutions.

7. The need to acknowledge and clarify the potential adverse social realities accompanying sickle cell. A clearly identified "enemy" allows for informed resistance.

In particular circumstances, as, for example, with parents in a trait by trait mating, or the birth of a child with sickle cell disease, or the exposure of nonpaternity, the relationship between the counselee and the counselor may continue over a period of months or years. The counselee needs to experience sustained caring from a person who will engage him in responsible review of the progress on the decisions made; for example, regular preventive health care for the infant with sickle cell disease; follow-through on a client's decision to avoid the risk of recurrence of sickle cell disease; and utilizing special services for individuals with sickle cell disease.

Determinants of Decision Making by Clients

A comment is in order on the goal of counseling for sickling disorders. It is commonly stated that the goal of such counseling is the prevention of the birth of individuals with sickle cell disease (Stamatoyannopoulos, 1974). It has been assumed that if prospective parents are presented the risk for their situation that they will make "informed decisions" leading to one of several choices: avoiding marriage between two individuals with the trait, refraining from reproduction in trait by trait marriages, or in the near future, obtaining prenatal diagnosis and, if necessary, a selective termination of pregnancy. The thrust of this chapter, however, has been that "informed decisions" may also lead to other goals, all of which conform to the definition of health for the individual or family, as presented at the outset of this chapter. It is likely that informed with facts clients frequently make decisions that least disturb their sense of personal or family equilibrium whether or not prevention of the disease is accomplished by the decisions.

Parental decisions that accept the risk of occurrence of sickle cell disease can be legitimate when made by self-aware parents. On the other hand, such decisions might represent parental fear, selfishness, or a limited insight about the psychosocial dynamics within a family. We might postulate that the specific decision a parent makes for or against preventing the birth of a child with sickle cell disease may be of less consequence than the long-term adaptive value of the decision for all members of that family. A high priority for research in this area is to quantify the perceived benefits of prospective counseling versus retrospective counseling apart from whether prevention per se is accomplished.

Times of psychosocial transition are occasions for reorganizing images of the self and of the external world. The occurrence of a painful situation, as for example when parents learn that they have produced a child with sickle cell disease, may elicit a judgment on the situation from each of the various selves within the individual parent. In so far as these judgments are concerned with perceived impediments to one's personal well-being there may emerge a set of conflicting evaluations that may paralyze effective decision making. Unaware of the many inner selves and their respective, sometimes conflicting, needs, the parent gives priority to that particular self or need that promises the easiest resolution of the stress or conflict. Such decisions may not be necessarily founded in reality.

Based on the principle that only what is named can be controlled, the self that feels angry at one's spouse or at God, the self that feels victimized, the self that feels guilt, the self that feels stigmatized and socially diminished, the self that denies any future responsibility for recurrence of sickle cell disease, must all be acknowledged by the client as real parts of the personality competing for principal authority over the crisis at hand (O'Connor, 1971). The astute counselor sets the stage for self examination so that the client can affirm the legitimacy of the many selves and can see the necessity of selecting the one that will creatively work with reality-based options for restoring personal well-being.

The model of reality therapy as advanced by Glasser (1965) appears to be particularly instructive at this point. In his view, relatedness and respect are essential universal human needs, and individuals vary in their ability to fulfill these needs. Given the psychosocial concomitants of sickle cell disease one might surmise that the client may suffer from a major assault against the fulfillment of both of these needs. Thus, beyond dealing with matters of biology, a primary responsibility of the counselor is to assist in restoring the fulfillment of relatedness and respect.

A review of research data, from other contexts, on the factors that shape the quality of the patient–doctor relationship and the effect of the latter on the quality of health care, indicates that empathy, nonpossessive warmth, and genuineness of the physician are significantly correlated with the effectiveness of therapy (Charney, 1972). The attention given at this point to the relationship between client and counselor is intended to emphasize its potentially determining role in decision making by the client. If it is accepted that the effectiveness of counseling is in part a function of the relationship and communication skills of the counselor, then research should be addressed to defining the qualifications required for the practice of sickle cell counseling.

References

Agle, D. P. Psychiatric studies of patients with hemophilia and related states. *Archives of Internal Medicine*, 1964, 114, 76–82.

Charney, E. Patient–doctor communication: Implications for the clinician. *Pediatric Clinics of North America*, 1972, 19, 263–279.

Dubos, R. The despairing optimist. *The American Scholar*, 1977, Autumn, 424–430.

Glasser, W. *Reality therapy*. New York: Harper and Row, 1965.

Headings, V. Alternative models of counseling for genetic disorders. *Social Biology*, 1976, 22, 297–303.

Headings, V. Associations between type of health profession and judgments about prevention of sickling disorders. *Journal of Medical Education*, 1976, *51*, 682–684.

Headings, V. and Fielding, J. Guidelines for counseling young adults with sickle cell trait. *American Journal of Public Health*, 1975, *65*, 819–827.

Langsley, D. G. Psychology of a doomed family. *American Journal of Psychotherapy*, 1961, *15*, 531–538.

Mischel, T. The concept of mental health and disease: An analysis of the controversy between behavioral and psychodynamic approaches. *The Journal of Medicine and Philosophy*, 1977, 2, 197–219.

Murray, R. F., Jr. Psychosocial aspects of genetic counseling. *Social Work in Health Care*, 1976, 2, 13–23.

O'Connor, E. *Our many selves.* New York: Harper and Row, 1971.

Phillips, J. R. Mental health and SCA: A psycho-social approach. *Urban Health*, 1973, 2, 36–40.

Powars, D. R. Natural history of sickle cell disease—The first ten years. *Seminars in Hematology*, 1975, *12*, 267–285.

Stamatoyannopoulos, G. Problems of screening and counseling in the hemoglobinopathies. In: *Birth defects: Proceedings of the fourth international conference on birth defects*, A. Motulsky, and W. Lenz, (Eds.). Amsterdam: *Excerpta Medica*, 1974, 268–276.

Tringo, J. L. The hierarchy of preference toward disability groups. The *Journal of Special Education*, 1970, *4*, 295–306.

Genetic "Russian Roulette": The Experience of Being "At Risk" for Huntington's Disease

12

Nancy Sabin Wexler

Huntington's disease, (HD) is an hereditary disorder of the central nervous system. It is transmitted through a single autosomal dominant gene with complete penetrance. Symptoms usually appear in adult life between the ages of 35 and 45. However, persons as young as 2 or as old as 80 have been known to develop the disorder. The disease is most often characterized by chronic progressive chorea and dementia, without remissions. The childhood form of HD, which affects 10% of cases and is inherited from the father 75% of the time, and some adult varients, are marked by rigidity rather than chorea. Psychoses and affective disorders as well as milder emotional disturbances are frequent either prior to or following the appearance of abnormal movements. Life expectancy after the onset of symptoms is on the order of 10 to 20 years for adults, 8 to 12 years for children. Death comes as a result of secondary infections, heart failure, or aspiration. There is no predictive test available and treatment is only marginally effective.

For the HD victim, the fatal determination is fixed at the moment of conception. Unknowing, the individual moves through life; the marked gene lies quiescent or its slow catabolic progress is masked by the forces of new cell birth. Then, at the peak of productivity, things go awry. At the stage when most individuals must face the transition from youth to middle age, the HD victim prepares for the passage from youth to death.

GENETIC COUNSELING
Psychological Dimensions

If the individual knows he or she is at risk, the years in anticipation of this change can be years of dread, of silent apprehension, of noisy emotional disarray, or of intense productivity. As is frequently the case with a late-onset genetic disorder for which there is neither a screening test nor treatment, individuals at risk are disease wise and doctor shy. They know the odds from an early age and often regard the genetic counselor with the same wary contempt the battlefield soldier shows for the journalist—ticking off in round numbers the daily toll of lives lost, reducing the human struggle to arid statistics. Nor is the psychological counselor seen as a source of refuge. Mental health workers are considered to be only for the mentally deranged while those at risk perceive themselves to be suffering from a physical threat.

As a clinical psychologist concerned with genetic diseases, I was interested in exploring how the two disciplines of psychology and genetics could pool their expertise to render a more comprehensive service to the client. If the genetic counselor is seen only as a purveyor of information, and the individual already is in possession of that information, he or she will not seek counseling. In order for counseling to be useful for well informed clients, both client and counselor must redefine their major task to be learning to cope with what is known. The genetic counselor or a psychotherapist familiar with genetics should be able to help the individual "work through" (in the psychoanalytic sense) the relevant facts. In doing so, the counselor must be sensitized to detect the subtle psychological effects that the state of genetic risk is likely to produce. It is my firm conviction that although individuals vary widely in their reactions to threat, there are still communalities of concern which cut across individual differences and these can be taught to counselors. In knowing approximately what to expect, the counselor is better able to listen, anticipate, probe, assure, and console.

In order to learn more about the inner world of an individual at risk for a serious genetic illness, I interviewed in-depth 35 persons at risk for HD. My respondents were 12 men and 23 women between the ages of 20 and 36. All had one parent, living or deceased, affected with HD. None had been diagnosed with HD or any other neurological disorder. All socioeconomic classes were represented, although most were in the middle or lower middle class. The mean level of education achieved was 14 years. The interviews, some conducted in my office, some in the respondents' homes, were open-ended and exploratory. What follows is a distillation of the main themes of these interviews as they emerged—the fears, griefs, and hopes of persons coping with an unusual life situation. They are the stories which would be told in the genetic counselor's office, if the door were open to them.

Reactions to HD Symptomatology

Every disease calls forth particular images and fears in its victims and potential victims. Cancer evokes the threat of pain and suffering; unpredictability is the hallmark of multiple sclerosis. For the person at risk for HD, the relevant metaphor is the time bomb. To be affected by HD had specific meanings for most of the at-risk individuals I spoke with, because of the nature of its symptomatology. The primary concerns for these people were the intellectual deterioration and personality changes wrought by the disease, the socially embarrassing choreiform movements, regressive problems such as incontinence, and, especially, the extreme dependency involved in becoming chronically ill.

All the at-risk individuals interviewed had known their affected parent and had watched that parent change and decline from a familiar, healthy person to someone somewhat unrecognizable, with bizarre movements, uncontrollable behavior, and slurred speech. For many of the interviewees these changes took place during the child's formative years, often leaving the child with a distorted understanding of the peculiar transformations that had claimed an often beloved parent.

In their adult years, these at-risk individuals still retained an image of the illness which they had conceptualized as children. Those who had been particularly frightened as children had especially sinister visions of the disorder as adults. In contrast, in families in which the ill parent was able to remain a functioning member of the family, even marginally, the children accepted the illness with greater equanimity. The nature of the children's early exposure to HD appeared to be critical in determining their adult adjustment to their own genetic risk.

For all these men and women at risk no matter how mature and well-adjusted they were to the presence of the illness in the family, the nature of HD symptomatology seemed to strike at the core of their physical and psychological self-esteem. The peculiarities caused by uncontrollable movements and mental deterioration became translated for many into a vision of a Frankensteinian monster, one who approaches others with affection but from whom mothers recoil in horror. Subjects spoke repeatedly of how "disgusting," "repulsive," "grotesque," "ugly and horrible" the HD patient becomes. There was a particular dread of losing bladder and bowel control. Some reported feeling nauseated at the sight of their ill parents. One 36-year-old father spoke poignantly of the horror of the anticipated bodily changes.

> It's an awful thing to look at your kids and wonder if some day they're going to look at you like some kind of monster . . . just to look in a

mirror and see yourself change like that. To look in people's eyes and
see how they're afraid . . . and they'd shy away from you and you'd
feel hurt. Years ago, you used to read how they'd burn people with
HD at the stake and things like that because they were possessed by
the devil. I can sure see why they would think so.

Despite the ghastliness of those visions, for all but two at-risk individuals
interviewed the most frightening aspect of HD was not the uncontrollable
movements but the loss of intellectual capacities. A 35-year-old woman
expressed the group's consensus, "You can live with jerkiness but you can't
live without your mind." Another woman had a recurrent dream that her
head was turning into oatmeal. Nearly all talked of "becoming a vegetable," "stagnating," "going crazy," "having your mind garbled," of not
being able to communicate, and of the terror of ending their lives in a
mental institution.

Then I saw my mother in the institution with other mental patients.
You can imagine what it was like for me to go in there. That's when
the severity of it really hit me. I realized it wasn't just like going off to
school and playgrounds, fine and everything. Seeing the bars on the
windows, I thought, "My God! Why do they need bars and everything" [woman, age 25].

Many at risk had parents who became paranoid and delusional as the
disease progressed. One man spoke of his horror and fear of mental illness
after seeing his aunt who was affected with HD. All the respondents
talked of personality changes and severe personality disturbances in the
affected parent, sometimes antedating the diagnosis of the disease by more
than 10 years.

Perhaps because most of the respondents were in the prime of their
productive years, with newly achieved independence, the threat of extreme
dependence on others as well as anticipated abandonment was another
anathema associated with the illness.

I worry about being a burden on my family financially. Here's a guy
who could've had everything but he's got somebody with HD. It'll
take all his money and all his time. I guess mostly I think of how he's
going to feel about it. This is why I want to fight; to fight for him.
That's horrible for the person who doesn't have it and loves this person
[woman, age 23].

The prospect of prolonged dependency and deterioration often made single
people despair of marrying while those married considered immediate divorce when they learned of their risk. The single people questioned
whether anyone could ever love and value them enough to want to share

that risk. A 22-year-old woman felt her anticipated loneliness to be one of the worst aspects of the disease.

> I guess, the thing I feel bad about on my part, the part I *really* dread, is having boyfriends see [my mother], 'cause I am very open about what it is and the fact that it's genetic and everything. And I think, wow, if they see how bad it is, it's just gonna be, "Forget it, baby." . . . It's not being terrified about having it sometime way in the future, like at the age of 35, it's always even when I was in high school, the thought of, oh, I'll never get married and, oh, I'll never be able to, like, it's never bothered me too much the idea of not being able to *bear* my own children, like I wouldn't mind adopting, but the thing of no one will marry me and the whole thing of being an old maid type of thing. It's really scared me more than just thinking about having the disease.

Those who were married wanted to protect themselves against the trauma of being left if they should become ill. Both groups fantasized taking active control either by not marrying or by divorcing; both felt that so great a burden of responsibility should not be inflicted on someone they loved.

> My problem is that all my aunts and uncles have divorced their HD victims. I think it's just awful! The first thing I said was that if you want a divorce, divorce me now because I'm not living alone when I'm sick! [Notice she says "when," not "if."] [woman, age 23]

One of the most frequently voiced fears is of choking and starving to death. Although this is a concern based on reality, it is as if the anticipated emotional abandonment *qua* starvation is also verbalized in these physical terms.

All of the interviewees were painfully aware that the disease is terminal, but for them termination comes not at the moment of death but at the moment of diagnosis. Most fantasize the period following diagnosis to be a prolonged and unproductive wait on death row. The optimism or pessimism of at-risk persons is directly related to the kind of care they perceive their ill parent to have received, regardless of the severity of the symptoms. When the sick parent is kept at home, or in a good nursing facility, active and a part of the community, the specter of the disease is not nearly as formidable.

None of the at-risk individuals mentioned feeling afraid of death, per se. On the contrary, death is often cited as a welcome relief from life with symptoms.

Q: What is the least frightening symptom of HD?

A: Probably that you die is the part that scares me the least. It's almost more human than the part where you live. I know it is a fatalistic outlook but I can't help it, sometimes. After seeing my aunt for seventeen years—she couldn't even roll over in bed—I definitely feel that dying is a relief [man, age 36].

Many subjects did not wish to wait passively as nature took its course. Approximately half the sample felt that they would seriously consider suicide as an option if and when they started to deteriorate. Most of these individuals came from families in which the ill parent had made at least one suicide attempt. (There were no completed suicides among the parents.) Others insisted that they would never consider suicide but they could understand how others might. One man, age 30, had what he called "death insurance." He had vowed to commit suicide when he was no longer able to function. If he was not aware of the severity of his deterioration, or was unable to carry out his plan, he had made a pact with his brother that each should kill the other, should it become necessary. Some subjects who did not consider suicide as a viable option expressed the wish to be institutionalized at the point when they were no longer able to lead useful lives.

Genetic Disease and Family Dynamics

It is impossible to understand fully the impact of HD on families without an appreciation of the complexities which its hereditary nature imposes. Every disease can arouse images of body damage and destruction; each can awaken fears of dependency and rejection. But only if the disorder is hereditary does an individual know the exact probability of contracting it. If the disease is an hereditary disorder of late onset, the individual has most likely witnessed the illness in parents or close relatives. Each individual must take the responsibility for risking passing on the disorder to future generations or refraining from procreation. Such hereditary illness can have repercussions throughout three or four generations simultaneously and have impact on parent–child identifications at each generational level. The history of the disease within the family has crucial ramifications for all those family members who are still genetically vulnerable. In fact, much of the working-through process which an at-risk individual must undergo to accept the illness is often expressed in terms of responses to other family members.

The first reaction which most individuals at risk reported when told of the presence of HD in their immediate family was an overwhelming concern and grief for the afflicted parent. If they already had children of their own, they also felt great sadness, protectiveness, and guilt toward the child. The most common immediate reaction was, "What have I done to my child!" Not only were they genuinely concerned for the welfare of the children, but the at-risk parents' own fears for themselves could be much more acceptably expressed in terms of anticipated calamity for the child.

> The fact that hit me the most—I used to cry whenever I looked at my son. I was afraid. Like, I was scared. I remember a real bad emptiness in my heart [woman, age 23].

Because of the late onset of HD and frequent inaccuracies in diagnosis, many of the people interviewed had not learned of the hereditary nature of their parents' illness until they themselves had had children. Six of the women were pregnant when they learned of the risk to themselves and to the unborn child. (Only two were in the first trimester and both decided to carry the baby to term.) One 28-year-old mother of two small children described her reaction on learning that her mother's disease was hereditary.

> I went through a bad depression for about two weeks . . . I'd sit there and cry because I'd think of how I might miss everything my mother missed. She never seen us married or have kids. She knows we have kids. I want to be a grandma . . . I told my husband I wanted a divorce so he could get out of the legal stuff—let the state take care of you. I'd tell him who I wouldn't want to watch the kids and who I would want. I wouldn't care if he'd get married again and have another woman to raise the kids so long as she loved them; so I would know they had a mother. I want to be home as long as possible but when the day comes, I want to be put in a nursing home . . . It was mainly the kids and how much of their lives I'd miss, depending on how old I was if and when I got it. I'd cry if I thought of any of their graduations or getting married. Anything like that would bring on a tear-jerk. And, of course, me not being there mainly for both of them. Then, after the two weeks I just snapped right out of it like I went into it. I've never given it another thought. I've done said everything like I wanted to.

In most normal families it is common for a child to hear, either in humor or in anger, "You're just like your mother, or father!" For the at-risk individual such a remark has an added impact. Whatever emotions at-risk persons experience toward the ill parent—tenderness, compassion, pity, disgust, resentment—may someday be the very feelings their own children experience toward them. As they watch their parents they watch themselves; all emotions rebound.

> What was upsetting was that here I'll be watching my Dad and maybe be watching myself. I felt I couldn't feel sorry for myself because I had to feel sorry for him. Yet here I was and nobody was going to feel sorry for me. I'd get mad at myself for being selfish [woman, age 25].

Frequently the person at risk becomes the confidante of the well parent who pours out grievances over the ill parent. The at-risk offspring is sometimes forced to mediate between the two. Often the child seeks to identify with the well parent and feels hostility for the sick parent for causing so much grief. Alternately, he or she may identify with the sick parent and experiences himself or herself as the potential recipient of the well parent's complaints. The child often urges the well parent not to be a "martyr"—not to sacrifice life and happiness because of the ill parent. Children frequently must listen to suicidal temptations of both parents. And yet while they say aloud that neither they nor their relatives should devote their whole lives to the sick, they usually are well aware that they are encouraging the same dreaded abandonment should they themselves become ill.

If parents with HD were particularly psychotic, violent, or unavailable, it becomes even more difficult for those at risk to cope with the prospect of getting the disease. They experience the possibility of possessing the HD gene as signifying that they would literally turn into their parent—a kind of cloning after birth. This fear seemed particularly powerful when the same-sexed parent was affected.

> I had the impression that HD was like what my mother was. I was ready to pack my bags and leave. If we wouldn't of stayed and talked to that social worker for two or three hours, I probably would have left. I really thought it was like what my mother was. I didn't know there was symptoms and all that stuff. I asked him if I was going to be like my mother was. When I found out I wasn't going to beat my kids, be mean and jealous, I calmed down. I didn't want to be like my mother to my kids; I'd sooner left [woman, age 28].

The dilemma of identification in a family affected by genetic disease has many complex ramifications. In the group interviewed, all of the at-risk individuals had had strained and disagreeable relationships with the ill parent for some time prior to the diagnosis of the disease. To most, the medical recognition that the parent was truly ill—apart from the hereditary nature of the illness—came as a welcome relief. The rage and disappointment they felt over the parent's inadequacy could thus be directed to something external—a sickness—for which neither parent nor child was to blame. The parent was not cruel, ill-tempered, or inconsistent because of a failure on the child's part, nor could the parent be held accountable for performing destructive and hostile acts. The child's guilt over murderous feelings harbored toward the parent was dissipated, but in its stead came fear. They reasoned that if HD caused behavior in the parent that was beyond control, might it not also cause the same behavior in the child if the child manifested the disease? This concern was especially felt by those individuals who witnessed a radical change in their parents from being loving and affectionate to being irritable and withdrawn or psychotic.

> But I think really, the thing that really scares me the most is I know, despite all my determination to hold myself together and be a pleasant person to be around, I fear that having the disease will make me lose that control and I'll turn into a shrew like my mother. And that will be what will alienate me from people. And that will be against my control, even though I won't want to do it. Like I see she does things that she doesn't want to do, but she can't help herself [woman, age 22].

The most reasonable resolution of the dilemma, and probably the most accurate, was for the individual at risk to perceive the ill parent as the victim of circumstances and background. At least the at-risk child did not share the parent's early environment. The real culprits thus become the grandparents and anger can be safely deflected from the parent. The grandparent is also to blame for passing on the gene, and both parent and child become hapless victims. Yet, while the parent has succumbed to his or her upbringing, the child fervently hopes to transcend environment and become quite different from the parent.

> When I first heard about it, I thought, "My God! She's gave me something else!!" I was bitter with my mother. Then, all of a sudden I started getting into her background and stuff [woman, age 23].

Remarkably few interviewees expressed conscious anger toward the parent who had given them this legacy. Compassion and grief were by far the most common feelings. It was considered in particularly bad taste to harbor hostility toward a parent who was already broken and ill. However, the child covertly disavowed the parent by trying to become as different as possible. Frequently, anger was turned against the self and expressed in depression. The following reaction of a young man, aged 20 when he learned of the disease, is quite typical.

I was angry and enraged [when I first found out about HD], you
know—gee, what a terrible thing! Just then, my mother died from
it. I grew up with it in my family. To think, I might have the same
thing someday. I don't even want to be sick a day with the flu or
anything. I haven't missed a day of work in three or four years. I just
try to stay as strong and healthy as I can. I think about it all the time.
Not all the time but like when I go to church on Sundays. I pray, you
know, give me strength and health. That's all I ask. I can take everything else from financial ruin to losing all my friends. As long as I've
got my health, I can come through. I don't like to be sick and a
burden on anybody. I just want to take care of my own life. I don't
want to be on welfare. That's a terrible thought. It could happen. It'd
be terrible if it does.

Q: When you think of HD, what do you think of?

A: I just kind of think your body'd waste away. You're just probably
tired all the time from shaking. That's a lot of physical exertion,
I'd imagine, moving all the time. It'd really take it out of you.
In a couple of years, you'd be exhausted. I try to keep my weight
up. I'm kind of over-weight for my size. I like that. I want to be
heavy and real strong. The charts recommend 140 lbs. for my size.
I weigh 175 lbs. That's fine– I weighed 200 lbs. a couple of years
ago when I first got married.

Q: Was your mother thin from HD?

A: Yeah. Your throat or anything doesn't function right. She'd try
to drink a Pepsi and choke on it.

Q: Did that scare you?

A: Oh gee!! People probably feel like committing suicide! I mean,
I wouldn't. I want to live as long as I can. I imagine if it comes to
that, if somebody's that sick, they'd want to get a whole bottle of
sleeping pills.

Q: Do you think you would?

A: I don't know. I'd hate to just be a vegetable. That's all you are.
You don't really function any more. Maybe you should be dead.
You'd probably be so far gone that it would be better to be dead.
It's hard to say. For myself, when I'm 35 years old it could happen then. Now I'm 24 and maybe I've only got ten more Christ-
mases to have good times in. Maybe I shouldn't feel that way. I
might be 60 like my other aunt. I sometimes wonder what families
are like that never have it.

Mr. M's initial reaction was one of anger and outrage at his mother.
He had had to put up with her severe emotional and physical problems
and now she had passed the threat on to him. However, resolution of
these feelings was aborted by the death of his mother and the feelings
were internalized. While it is true that most HD patients become emaciated
and cachexic, Mr. M seems to fear the total annihilation of his body.
It is as if the internalized feelings of rage and disappointment will
dissolve his very physical being. He tries to counteract this anxiety with

exaggerated weight and solidity. If this defense should fail, he contemplates suicide, particularly by "eating" an overdose of pills. Mr. M acts as if he might wake up one morning when he is 35 and find that his life is over. He hopes desperately to be one who escapes and then wishes, rather wistfully, to be quit of the whole concern.

Whether or not a person feels destined either to develop or to escape the disease has repercussions in attitudes towards siblings. A surprisingly large number of those at risks felt emotionally convinced, regardless of what they intellectually knew, that at least one of their sibship must develop the disease. They considered that feeling free of the disease was tantamount to inflicting it on a relative. One woman thought herself a "marked target" because she was the youngest of three and her sibs appeared to be healthy. A very thoughtful young man felt he should get the disease because his sibs all had children and he did not.

Respondents frequently expressed the feeling that they could be free of HD only by paying some price. One woman volunteered: "Spare me and I'll be a good Samaritan and care for the rest." Others make more modest requests; they wish only to be left for last. The notion of hoping that the entire family escape altogether is considered almost too greedy to be expressed aloud: God punishes hubris. One 25-year-old woman's dream graphically illustrates this point.

> I have always had nightmares. Now, the fear in my dreams is that I'm being followed by someone. The last one I had was where my friends and relatives were in a big room, a big house. There was this one man. I could see him but I couldn't warn anyone. He would go up to them and stick pins in them. When he stuck enough pins in you, you died. He was eventually going to come back to me but he was going to leave me until the end and get all my friends and relatives first. I couldn't stop him from doing it.

"Waiting for Godot"

One of the most psychologically unacceptable notions which confronts the individual at risk is to be the passive victim of a totally random genetic accident. One 28-year-old woman described being at risk as "playing Russian roulette with a two-barreled gun and somebody else's hand on the trigger." Subjects perceived their lives and their universes as conforming to the laws of cause and effect; true randomness was either unacceptable or unassimilatable on more than an intellectual level.

Surely they are not unique in this way of thinking. In general parlance we speak of "chance" in the context of being "lucky" or "unlucky"—a personal attribute which, as it were, controls chance and mitigates against randomness. When an individual has been the victim of a violent crime, others often respond with accusations instead of sympathy. The victim is considered to have covertly incited the crime through some careless or inappropriate behavior. Even the victim often feels ashamed and self-recriminatory. The advantage to this way of thinking is that the crime can thus be attributed to a specific action that then can be avoided by others in the future. If disaster, either natural or man-made, is truly random, then we are all and at all times vulnerable. Some, like Mr. M, manage their fears by turning to a higher order of control and explanation in the medium of religion. God can be influenced through prayer and good deeds. If He should choose to inflict the disease, then it is not randomly assigned but made meaningful through God's will.

On an unconscious level, many of the at-risk respondents view the transmission of HD in the context of crime and punishment. This feeling is especially fostered in families where the illness is regarded as a family curse and not discussed. To them, it is truly that "the sins of the fathers are visited upon the sons." Sometimes the "crime" stems from anger toward the ill parent or from the forbidden wish that another relative inherit the disease instead. A few subjects communicated a Kafkaesque sense of bewilderment at their feelings of guilt. A 20-year-old girl stated this explicitly;

> It seems that so many things have gone bad in my life that with this HD thing, well, it almost seems like I must have done something wrong somewhere to deserve all this.

If an at-risk person is violent, moody, suspicious, jealous, or disagreeable, it is considered as an ominous sign that the disease is developing. The disease is sometimes considered as just punishment for these unpleasant traits. At-risk individuals often develop complicated and constant systems of monitoring themselves in mood and movement. They continually check their hands, gait, memories, and emotions, not really to identify the disorder if it occurs, but in order to exert control over what may be happening to them.

> Sometimes I hold my hands out to see if my fingers wiggle . . . I just hope they aren't shaking and I can control them. Usually I'm really cool about it. It just seems like maybe tense people are nervous people and it looks like a mild case of it. They get scared that way . . . I guess, maybe, I always try to walk straight with a good posture. I try to see if I shake. I don't know what it'd feel like. Sometimes I can feel my heart beating in my body. I imagine everybody gets that. Some-

times my heart will beat so strong I can feel my fingers move with each beat. I guess maybe that I watch my face . . . Sometimes when people are waiting they'll cross and uncross their legs and shake them. I try not to do that and hold perfectly still [male, age 24].

Shortly after learning of his at risk status, one artist in his mid-20s wrote a play in which the hero was also at risk. This fictional character would stand in front of the mirror for hours practicing facial grimaces, rehearsing, and thus accustoming himself through practice with the person he might become. Through this double distancing of hero-within-a-play, the author was trying to gain active mastery over the disease. He would go out and claim it, as it were, rather than passively wait for the illness to overtake him. This same man said rather ruefully that he envied his wife "her right to be clumsy." His use of the word "right" implicitly suggests that he considers himself to be deprived of his "rights," that is, to be punished.

Considering that most at-risk individuals were most frightened by the psychological aspects of HD, it is not surprising that many tried to influence the course and even the onset of the disease through the use of their minds. Almost every subject spoke of staving off the effects of the disease through "strength of will."

My mother would say, "With your heritage, I wouldn't get mad like that." In other words, don't get mad 'cause you'll go crazy. She would say things like: "Watch out . . . don't do this or don't do that, don't feel, don't trust people, they'll leave you." The people that got left— they all got the disease. I got messages like: you have no right to your feelings. You can't feel angry. If you feel scared you'd better hide it. Don't ever cry. All of them had to do with the disease. Those were all heavy, strict injunctions on feelings. My mother's injunctions were that if you control your feelings well enough, be in charge of yourself at all times, then you can control your mind and you won't get this [woman, age 23].

The "power of positive thought" is a relief from the terrifying help-lessness of passivity for many at risk. Its liability, however, is that the individual becomes responsible for the presence or absence of the disease. To develop the illness means failure of control or failure of faith.

I've made my prayers and asked to not get it. I have strong faith but it's not that strong in that area. I have really strong faith. I can ask a prayer and sit there and wait. But this thing is so powerful that I need a stronger faith. Maybe, eventually, I will get that. Faith might save me. You can ask a prayer but if you haven't got faith, then it won't get answered [woman, age 36].

Subjective Prediction: Second Guessing the Unknown through Magic

Although the laws of probability predict that approximately half the individuals interviewed will eventually develop this disease (disregarding sampling bias possibly introduced through the use of volunteers), three-quarters of the respondents felt certain that they would become afflicted. Nearly all those who felt that they would *not* develop HD as well as those who thought they would, expressed magical and highly unrealistic reasons to support their beliefs. Only a very few of those who were convinced that they would remain healthy gave as evidence that they were in their mid-30s and had been symptom-free on repeated neurological check-ups. One woman in this latter group was afraid to put her optimism into words, however, for fear it would be "bad luck." Others in the group who felt they had "escaped" gave far less reasonable explanations.

Typical of their responses was that of one man who was sure he would escape the disease because he had "always been lucky." He also considered himself to be somewhat psychic. (This man had been told by his older sister that every third child manifested HD; naturally, he was the third child.)

Those who felt certain they did harbor the defective gene had equally magical and unrealistic explanations: they had always been unlucky at lotteries, or everything else bad had happened in their lives. One woman felt that "the genes would have been stronger in the first conception" and that as the eldest she would certainly get it. A rather more powerful and subtle argument was that they looked or acted like their affected parents, that is, were nervous, moody, irritable, etc.

Probably the most common dynamic operating in those who felt convinced they would develop HD was the attempt to combat the passivity of waiting through active control. As part of that activity there was also a frequently implied magical belief that if they "sacrificed" themselves to the disease they would be rewarded by being spared. Like Abraham with Isaac, their devotion to their siblings, their humility, their unselfishness, and their willingness to suffer was being tested and at the last moment they would be reprieved. On an unconscious level, genetic randomness is seen as mediated by a moral universe. Consciously, many subjects expressed the feeling that if they expected and prepared for the worst they could only be surprised by something positive.

Predictive Tests

All of the subjects firmly believed that a predictive test should be developed, regardless of their own hesitations to utilize it. Approximately two-thirds of the subjects said, with varying degrees of conviction, that they would take a predictive test. Reactions ranged from thoughtful realism to bravado; all acknowledged that they would be terrified to avail themselves of the test. Some subjects responded as if they felt they ought to want to know, while others were adamant about the importance of being able to plan realistically for their future. For the latter, the ambiguities of limbo were psychologically more difficult to bear than the certain knowledge that they were carrying the HD gene. All suggested that counseling be made available with thep redictive test. In this way subjects and their families could be aided in coping with emotional reactions and other repercussions both before and after taking the test.

Those who would not take a predictive test were vociferous in their wish not to know their genetic inheritance. Some said they would take a test only if there were successful ways of treating the disease. They clung to their 50–50 chances and would not want to risk losing them. One 23-year-old woman best expressed the feelings of many at risk, as follows:

Q: If there was an accurate predictive test available, would you take it?
A: Really, no, but knowing myself I probably would.
Q: Why?
A: For the fact that it's a step forward. For the fact that if it's a crisis, God, get it over with. I'm so tired of wondering. If they would tell me that I wasn't going to get it, they could take my arm off! What if they do tell you you've got HD, how do you live with that? Like, if they were to say to me today, "You're going to get HD when you are 30," do you know what every day would be like? Every day would not be a real life. . . . I just couldn't live with that. Now, at least I have a 50–50 chance; knowing and not knowing. I can live with that. Now, I have optimism. Then it would be real.
Q: Do you think scientists ought to develop such a predictive test?
A: It would be good for science to have a predictive test but it wouldn't be good for the HD victim. Can you imagine knowing that there's some place you can just walk into? Every day, that would prod your mind, "I'm going. I'm going. Just for the sake of science, I'm going. For the sake of knowing, I'm going. I can't stand it anymore." Then all of a sudden, having somebody tell you you're going to have HD. I think this would prey on their minds and everybody would probably go. But they really wouldn't want to.

Family Planning and Prediction

One-fourth of the at risk individuals interviewed had children after learning of the hereditary nature of the disease. Most subjects had already established families before learning of the genetic nature of their parent's illness. Of this latter group, the majority claimed that had they known, they would have chosen to adopt children. Many of those married without children, however, wanted their own. There were indications that several in the group with children had known at some level that the disease was hereditary, but did not acknowledge this awareness until after their children were born.

> When we were kids, we didn't know what was wrong with them but we knew all three of them were alike. They walked alike. They smoked alike. They moved alike. We promised each other that if we ever got like that we were going to come and kill each other. We knew it was something bad [woman, age 28].

Only two childless subjects, a 24-year-old male and 25-year-old female, had been sterilized; others were sterilized after creating a family. Over half of the single people at risk had decided not to have their own biological children, unless this decision prevented them from marrying the person of their choice. Many in this group were deeply concerned about the impact their decision not to bear children would have on their marriageability. They felt that being at risk in itself made them defective and denying their future spouse natural children made them even less desirable as marriage partners. Yet to be single and forced to cope alone with HD was a prospect filled with horror. An exceptionally attractive 22-year-old woman articulated one of the primary concerns of persons at risk.

Q: Do you think that maybe you turn away some of the men who are interested in you?
A: Well, I have had this feeling. When I meet somebody who's super intelligent, super good-looking—this guy should have kids; this guy should propagate his kind. This guy wouldn't want to adopt. I do think about that. And having the guy smarter than me is an absolute requirement and that's something that I'm not willing to compromise. But having the guy not too good looking is one thing I even search for. Number one, because then he won't feel like, oh, I'm so good looking I've got to have a whole bunch of me's running all over the world. And also, I feel like I'd be able to hold him easier, be able to trap him easier. Which is kind of a whole bad syndrome that I'm

in . . . I think, wow, since I'm at risk, I'm less attractive as a possible mate, so I've got to compromise somewhere, give up something of my desires for a mate. So, I'm not willing to give up personality or strength or the intellectual capacity, so the one thing that's left is looks. So I'm sort of hunting for some ugly guy (laugh). I think the worst part is that no one will marry me and I'll have to be alone. I guess it's the fear of having HD and being alone at that point, and being abandoned by all my so-called friends. But that could happen with a spouse, too. I guess that's why having a sister is a real comfort, because I don't think she'd abandon me.

To marry and have children means to these individuals to lead a normal life. It strengthens the normal denial that anything may be wrong. If people at risk choose to forego having children or choose to adopt, they are acting as if the illness were a certainty. The woman who had a tubal ligation rather than risk passing on the gene felt she was "damned if she did and damned if she didn't." If she tried to accept the fact that she had been sterilized, it meant to her that she had HD; if she thought that she might remain healthy, she could not bear the thought that she had had herself sterilized for no reason. It was extremely hard for her to act in one circumstance as if she would have HD and take appropriate precautions and still maintain the belief that she could as likely be well. Childless subjects feel that they are faced with the choice of guilt or self-deprivation. To alter one's life to the extent of foregoing natural children means to acknowledge genuinely the reality of being at risk. Many genetic counselors report being surprised and disappointed by how many at-risk individuals have children. These counselors fail to realize the symbolic and magical significance of the child as an insurance of the parent's continuing health. It is also true that many at-risk persons are being asked to give up one "route to immortality" through their children at the same time that they are coping with their own potential death. If genetic counseling involved more in-depth counseling over a greater length of time, perhaps more at-risk couples would choose to adopt. The fact that many adoption agencies consider a person at risk not a suitable parent creates additional complications and emotional stresses.

Learning to Live in Limbo

There is an existentialist maxim that one cannot be really free until one has come to terms with one's own death. In their own words and through their actions, many of these at-risk individuals expressed this feeling: "If I can't live quantity, then I'll have lived quality." For some, of course, the potentiality of a reduced life span became translated into a constriction of their current lives and an unwillingness to take risks.

> We're always talking new house. I don't know if it's good or bad but I always turn him off. In my opinion, we're living comfortably now and I can't see moving into a new house. I'm afraid to take a step into the future. I just can't talk about the future because I don't really believe in the future. I'm just living now. When somebody talks of the future, I just turn myself off. I don't believe I'm going to be part of it. If it's going to happen, I don't know how because I'm afraid to make a move [woman, age 28].

Most of the subjects were not as reluctant as this woman to plan for and dream of the future. All, however, shared her feeling of urgency, her emphasis on living for the here and now.

> I'd say I started feeling an urgency to live; do everything right now and not wait for everything. I think I lived in the future a lot. It made me feel more pushed to finish school. That was always a dream of mine. None of my relatives had ever been to college [woman, age 33].

> I mean, it's always in the back of your mind. The least little back-slide you have, you think about it. That's why I get depressed sometimes. If something doesn't turn out as I expect, I think maybe there won't be another chance. I don't think like that very often. Sometimes I do [woman, age 36].

> I feel there is no way I can escape it. I have to make my mark by a certain period of time. I have to do something very important with my life and not waste it. There has always been a sense of urgency in absolutely everything I've done [man, age 30].

> There are times when I think about it but not when I'm dancing. I think that I love to dance so much. I dance every day—I just dance. I think about this—what am I going to do if I do have it? Because I really love to dance. I love to just be moving around. I've just kind of felt that I've got to get it all out of my system. If I can just dance now while I can and try everything I want to try [woman, age 25].

Many of the respondents felt that they had gained an enriched perspective on life in living more for the here and now. They questioned their previous values and felt more able to concentrate their energies on activities and relationships that were meaningful to them. An intensified wish to "make a mark early in life" often led to creative and productive work and, in fact, an increased willingness to take risks. Five of the women interviewed had gone back to school or had taken jobs which brought them a great deal of pleasure and pride. All of them claimed that the courage to make these changes in their lives stemmed directly from the knowledge that they were at risk. None of those interviewed wished to squander their lives but rather, in their own fashion, each voiced the desire to "see life whole and see it clear."

Psychotherapeutic Suggestions

Almost every respondent in this study could benefit from short- or long-term counseling focused on coping with HD in the family. When at-risk persons first learn of their own risk or when they come for genetic counseling, there is often so much substantive information to be imparted that there is not enough time for discussing emotional reactions. There is also an initial shock that shields against problems that arise later. None of the individuals interviewed had had any counseling other than that provided sporadically and on a volunteer basis by the Hereditary Disease Foundation, the Committee to Combat Huntington's Disease, or the National Huntington's Disease Association. For most, their only contact with a knowledgeable professional was their parents' physician. Genetic counselors, they felt, focus only on issues of procreation and are not available over a long period to discuss problems as they change over time. Given the mobility of our society, perhaps families should be encouraged to form an institutional alliance, a transference to an informed and responsive genetic or psychological clinic rather than only to an individual.

Based on my experience working with persons at risk for HD the following counseling suggestions are offered. Although they were developed with a specific population in mind, it is hoped that they will be relevant to many counseling situations in which a genetic illness is involved.

1. *Listen.* Many at risk individuals find that their spouses, their immediate family, or their relatives are too involved, too frightened or too guilty to really listen. Most persons at risk do not want to frighten their families with their concerns. They also especially do not want other family members to watch them for symptoms.

2. *Do not minimize the gravity of their concern but offer realistic hope.* Because of their own difficulties in coping with the risk situation, family members often brush aside the at risk person's concerns, scoff at them, or offer magical-omnipotent solutions. Spouses are notorious for such statements of denial as: "Don't worry, honey, I won't let you get it," or "It can't happen to us." Although optimism is a must, it can also be frightening to the at-risk person to feel that the spouse cannot afford to think that it *could* happen to them. It means that the disease is truly too terrible to think about. Frequently the spouse has a realistic appraisal

of the situation but a conspiracy of silence regarding the disease grows between the couple because each does not want to frighten the other. A counselor can be extremely helpful in guiding the individual or the couple toward a realistic appraisal of the disorder, acknowledging the reality of their concerns, giving hope, and thereby demonstrating that the illness can be reasonably discussed without anybody coming to grief.

3. *The fact that anyone might die suddenly in an accident is not effective consolation.* Many people will try cheering persons at risk with statements like, "Don't worry about it, you could step off the curb and get hit by a truck." It is true, but not truly helpful. Most people at risk are concerned about the process of dying, not with death itself. It is more valuable to stress the quality of life, both in health and sickness. In this case getting HD is only a 50% risk, but many at risk make themselves 100% miserable worrying while they are healthy. Much of their apprehension concerns the treatment they will receive should they become ill. Many have retained childhood visions of a "lunatic" parent, strapped in bed, with no medication. The counselor should emphasize the new drugs which are now available, new health care insurance which is pending, better nursing facilities, increased awareness of HD in the medical community, and the efficacy of physical and psychological therapy in staving off some of the most frightening symptomatology. If the state of being ill is seen as less frightening, anxiety will decrease. Remind individuals that a 50/50 probability means as great a chance that they will *not* get HD as that they will. The likelihood that the disease will appear also begins to decline after the '40s.

4. *The counselor should remember that the state of being at risk is qualitatively different from the state of knowing definitively either that one will be sick or healthy.* The ambiguous condition of 50% risk is extremely difficult to maintain in one's mind, if not impossible. In practice, a 50–50 risk translates to a 100% certainty that one will or will not develop the disease, but the certainty changes from one to the other from moment to moment, day to day, month to month. It can be helpful to discuss this phenomenon with counselees so that they know that fluctuations in their convictions are a normal part of the coping process.

5. *"Symptom Searching."* Every at-risk individual is continually on the alert for any suspicious signs of the disorder. Even if they deny that they check themselves if asked directly, many will give examples in the course of general conversation of such self-diagnoses. Every time an at-risk person trips, stumbles, mumbles, falls, forgets, has a car accident, gets enraged, or gets divorced, the specter of HD is aroused for themselves and for others. Many are so hyperalert that they make themselves uncoordinated, frightening themselves even more. There are at-risk individuals

who practice walking on lines, walking on curbs, controlling their hand-writing, controlling their speech, touching their fingers to their noses, and even rehearsing Serial Sevens! Others practice how it would be to have HD. Occasionally they frighten themselves by not knowing when the practice stops and the real thing begins. They try to master the disease through activity in the same way that people who very much fear "going crazy" play "being crazy." Some at risk will imitate mannerisms of the affected parent as an identification with that parent. It can be extremely reassuring to explain that all who are at risk "symptom-seek" and that most feel convinced that they will develop the disease. The counselor should teach the individual about psychological defenses and how they may be operating, as well as about normal muscular tics and twitches such as myoclonic bursts and normal psychological lapses, including especially normal forgetfulness.

6. *Differentiate HD from the rest of the environment.* Freud once said that if you cordon off one portion of a city and tell the police they cannot enter, you can be sure where to find all the criminals. The prospect of having HD can feed into every conflict; and each problem can be interpreted in terms of HD, rendering it relatively hopeless in the eyes of the individual. For some it may be easier to lay the blame with HD rather than face vulnerabilities, failures, or weaknesses that have nothing to do with the disease. Work with the individual to differentiate realistic concerns regarding the illness from fantasied concerns and from conflicts which are unrelated. Most problems stem from the usually disrupted environments in which these people have been raised.

7. *Relieve guilt.* The counselor should be attuned to any expressions of conscious or unconscious guilt on the part of the client. Often the guilt is pervasive and extends both toward the parents and toward the children. Guilt may be over anger toward and neglect of the parent, over envy of an obviously well sibling, over the desire to bear one's own children, and so forth. In particular, the counselor should try to make explicit the common belief that good or bad behavior will have an influencing effect on whether or not the individual develops the disease. Often the environment conspires with this belief: A 12-year-old girl at risk was told by a police matron that she had "better behave or she would get what her mother had."

8. *Just as prediction is usually foremost in the minds of the at-risk individual, it is often foremost in the mind of the counselor: Will this person develop HD?* In my opinion, most HD patients do not get diagnosed until approximately 3 to 10 years or more after the initial mani-festations of the disorder. This does not mean that they are unaware of the disease prior to the diagnosis. A well-trained observer may be able

to detect subtle neurological, cognitive, and psychological cues long before the person with HD feels it necessary (or is pushed) to be diagnosed. What have been thought in the past to be socio-psychological indicators of neurological pathology may be, in fact, indicative of a psychological reaction to a perceived change in performance, but should never be taken as sufficient indications of the disease in and of themselves. Extreme pain, anger, and/or an ill-advised decision to have children can result from an inaccurate prediction of future events and counselors should avoid speculation, even if they are optimistic. If, on the other hand, the counselor feels convinced that the individual is not manifesting any signs of the illness *at that moment in time,* it can be very encouraging for the client to hear this opinion. Above all, the counselor should be empathic and respond to the concerns of the client as they are expressed.

Genetic Counseling and Cancer[1]　　13

H. T. Lynch
Patrick M. Lynch
Jane F. Lynch

In recent years there has been an avalanche of information pertaining to genetic or familial diseases and to early detection of such diseases through amniocentesis, fetoscopy, or fetal biopsy. More dramatically, rhetorical questions are being asked by members of families which manifest hereditary disorders on the general subject of "What can we do about the family curse?" These concerns have infiltrated the lay press to such an extent that the typical patient is no longer reluctant to probe his physician about the facts and implications of his family history. Thus, the average practicing physician is becoming accustomed to patients' concerns which deal directly with problems traditionally considered to be in the specialized domain of medical genetics. The patient expects and indeed deserves an accurate and reasonable answer to his queries about how his family history might influence his own susceptibility to a particular disorder. The patient should be informed fully regarding the likely prognosis and disposition of his own medical problem and should receive an explanation of how the risk for the particular condition might be transmitted to and manifested in his children. A positive family history of a particular disorder may also modify the physician's choice of diagnostic and treatment measures and could in certain circumstances lead to cancer prevention.

Unfortunately, the bulk of currently practicing physicians are not sufficiently experienced in the discipline of medical genetics to be able to delve into many of these genetic counseling problems with the necessary

[1] Partial support for this was given by the Fraternal Order of Eagles.

221

expertise and depth that may be required. The majority of physicians who graduated from medical school more than 2 decades ago will have had only a very limited exposure to medical genetics. Therefore, unless they have availed themselves of the recent abundance of literature on the subject, their knowledge may be too limited to provide comprehensive genetic counseling to their patients. Recent graduates of medical schools have been more thoroughly exposed to medical genetics since this discipline is now included in most medical school curricula. The World Health Organization (1969) has recognized the importance of the manpower problem and has recommended increased training of medical personnel in medical genetics, with particular emphasis on genetic counseling. We subscribe wholeheartedly to this admonition.

The purpose of this chapter is to focus attention upon one facet of genetic counseling, namely the specialized area of cancer genetics where a variety of hereditary disorders have placed patients at markedly elevated risk for cancer. Some of these risks have been derived empirically. Others have followed simple genetic inheritance patterns. Because of the genetic heterogeneity in many of these disorders, we now know that it is a superficial exercise to speak, for example, of the "genetics of breast cancer" without paying particular heed to the problem of clinical variation shown by tumor association in this disease, as evidenced by the multiple putative genotypes (Lynch, Guirgis, Brodkey, Lynch, Maloney, Rankin, & Mulcahy, 1976). In order to facilitate applications of genetic counseling methods to the broad range of hereditary cancer associated syndromes, the authors will present briefly their own philosophy, objectives, and experiences in genetic counseling, with an emphasis upon the psychological and social needs of the patient.

Cancer as a Unique Genetic Counseling Problem

The problems encountered in the genetic counseling of cancer may differ from those involved in noncancerous diseases. In the former situation, the counselee is frequently an adult who has already had his or her desired number of children and is past the usual age of procreation. Such an individual may hold himself responsible for the increased cancer risk to his progeny and feel guilty for it. This problem becomes vividly clear when, as is so often the case in cancer genetics, an autosomal dominant gene is segregating in the family. Obviously then, if the parent has had cancer or is known to be at exceedingly high risk for harboring the deleterious gene, such guilt feelings are compounded by the acute concern for continued personal well-being. This is unlike the situation involving recessive disorders where, although the risk to children may be high, the heterozygous parent is usually in no personal danger of manifesting the disease. Exceptions to this may exist in heterozygous carriers of the gene for ataxia telangiectasia and Fanconi's aplastic anemia (Lynch, 1976).

The late age of onset of certain forms of cancer is particularly problematic in that the patient may have to wait many years before he knows whether or not he will be affected with the disease. This wait-and-see necessity may itself be disconcerting and frightening. What do the persons at risk do about marriage, procreation, and other life decisions? If they wait until they are beyond the age of greatest genetic cancer risk, and decide they are one of the fortunate 50% of unaffected offspring, then it may be too late to marry and have children. This is the critical problem in dominant disorders with late onset. Other issues may pertain to their career goals and how they should be pursued in light of the cancer risk under which the patient must labor.

A considerable body of literature (Day, 1966) and our own experiences have shown that profound emotional responses may be shown by the entire family unit (including spouses) once a diagnosis of cancer has been made and the risk to other family members becomes known. These responses are modified significantly by the type of malignant neoplasm involved, its age of onset, clinical course (which may vary from complete survival or cure to that of a rapid and fulminating demise, such as occurs in certain forms of acute leukemia, malignant melanoma, and bronchogenic carcinoma), and the degree of financial stress which the family sustains. Not only may a number of family members become affected, but on occasion the occurrences in a given sibship may follow in rapid succession, proving catastrophic to the family unit.

A vicious circle may be engendered in which the family members manifest anxiety, fatalism, denial, and even accusation directed toward the spouse, parents, or other family members who have "caused the disease among us." In certain cases, the emotional response is directed against the self, expressed as the need for punishment, due to feelings of blame for having transmitted the cancer risk to one's offspring.

In certain situations, the patient's peer group may compound the already discouraging situation. For example, in cosmetically disfiguring disorders such as dominantly inherited neurofibromatosis or the multiple mucosal neuroma syndrome (Lynch, 1972), the community may adopt an untoward attitude which leads to a repugnant response, not only against afflicted patients, but against relatives of the particular patient (Krush, Krush, & Lynch, 1965). In short, the counselor must be fully aware of community reaction as a factor in the psychological response of the family.

A Colon-Cancer-Prone Family

The following discussion reviews an attitude survey which was conducted as part of a medical genetic study of a family prone to site-specific colon cancer in association with occasional solitary adenomatous polyps of the colon (Lynch, Lynch, Harris, Lynch, & Guirgis, In press). Although colon cancer predisposition was transmitted as a dominant factor and the typical target site was the colon (more particularly the cecum), the pre-neoplastic state was only manifested by solitary colon polyps and even these did not appear in all patients.

Twenty-six members of this kindred who resided in or near a large county in northwestern Iowa were interviewed. They ranged in age from 32 to 78 years. Four of the family members had already had at least one surgical procedure for colon cancer and another seven were at high risk for colon cancer by virtue of having an affected parent. Since the unusual clinical findings in the family suggested that early diagnosis and treatment would likely be a problem, one purpose of the field visit was to assess each relative's existing knowledge of the familial cancer predisposition, determine how this awareness affected, for better or worse, any given member's attitude toward his or her own prospects for developing cancer, and how this attitude was translated into action or inaction in terms of requests for cancer screening examinations.

Most of the family members had a general idea of the extent of cancer in the family, suspected that there was a familial predisposition to colon cancer (although this was generally characterized as a family "weakness"), and typically felt themselves to be at increased risk. Interestingly, those persons having an affected parent or sibling did seem to be more concerned about their own risk than those patients who did not have an affected parent. Furthermore, the older, unaffected, at risk individuals correctly intuited that for some reason they were "over the hump" or beyond the age where they would expect to have been affected (modified life-tables showed highest colon cancer risk to be between ages 40 and 60).

Unfortunately, this was about as far as the insights extended. Awareness of some ill-defined risk notwithstanding, most of the individuals we evaluated stated that they would not go to their family physician for a cancer screening examination unless and until symptoms were present. This delay phenomenon has been extremely well documented in other cancer-prone families (Brasher, 1954). None of the persons who had a close relative die of colon cancer felt less confident about the ability of their physicians to deal with the problem. To a great extent the repeated cancer occurrences were considered a matter of fate and while early detection was felt to improve a patient's chances somewhat, it could not guarantee prolonged survival. In short, despite the fact that family members did not appear to be so concerned about their cancer risk that they would diligently seek consultation from their physicians, all were quite interested in learning more regarding the risks to themselves and their children, what the possible manifestations of early cancer might be, and what could be done in the future to detect colon cancer in its earliest stages. In our view, these considerations comprise the rudiments of genetic counseling.

In addition to describing the nature of the syndrome as it was then understood by us, family members who were at risk were informed that a similar discussion of pertinent findings would also be forwarded to their family physicians. This was in fact done and several of the physicians expressed their appreciation for having been informed of clinical features to be searched for in their patients. Indeed, one of our recommendations was to proceed with total colectomy (prophylactic) on those patients who had already experienced colon cancer and who had had a hemicolectomy. Two patients in this particular category have now undergone total prophylactic colectomies and a third is planning to have one performed in the future. Significantly, an occult carcinoma of the cecum was histologically verified in the resected colon of one of these two patients. On follow-up, each patient appeared to be satisfied with the decision to have prophylactic colectomy performed, that is, each has resumed normal bowel function following ileo-rectal anastomosis and none have had second thoughts on the subject. However, it must be reemphasized that these patients had already had a colon carcinoma and were therefore reasonably certain to have been carriers of the deleterious gene. So far in this family, no individuals who are simply at statistically high risk (having a colon cancer-affected parent) have undergone prophylactic colectomy, perhaps in part due to the above-mentioned belief in acting only upon symptoms of actual disease.

Family Management and Education

Since this family is still under investigation, a determination of the number of family members who have evidence of colon polyps but who have not been affected by colon cancer is incomplete. Given the lack of distinguishing pre-cancerous physical stigmata we feel that available diagnostic procedures, including colonoscopy, proctosigmoidoscopy, and barium enema may be inadequate in identifying those patients who will eventually be affected by cancer. Markers such as indices of proliferation of colonic mucosal cells may eventually aid in this problem (Lipkin & Deschner, 1976). Marker systems might also prove useful in diagnosing other familial colon cancer-prone syndromes and perhaps sporadic or nonfamilial varieties of colon cancer susceptibility as well. Despite the fact that such tests may at this time be considered only experimental, strongly positive test findings, as evidenced by an increased cellular proliferation index, could then be incorporated into the genetic counseling process.

We consider it to be of paramount importance that a balance be struck between the research plan and experimental testing described above and day-to-day clinical management of a large, extended, cancer-prone kindred. Where reliable clinical features (multiple polyps in familial polyposis coli) or biochemical markers (such as elevated calcitonin in Sipple's syndrome) are present, detailed family studies may not be required for full elucidation of familial trait. In such circumstances, all that may be necessary before counseling of the patient takes place are: (a) a firm diagnosis; (b) knowledge that two or more family members are affected in order to distinguish familial from sporadic occurrences (fresh germinal mutation can never be excluded); and (c) an awareness of the mode of transmission of the trait. Unfortunately, even in these situations, sound management of the family as a whole has been the exception rather than the rule (Lynch, 1969). In contrast to the above, there are many autosomal dominantly inherited cancerous and pre-cancerous syndromes which lack recognizable clinical signs, such as the Cancer Family Syndrome (Lynch & Krush, 1971), the familial association of breast and ovarian cancer (Lynch, Guirgis, Albert, Brennan, Lynch, Kraft, Pocekay, Vaughns, & Kaplan, 1974), and the colon cancer syndrome described here. In these vertically transmitted syndromes, determination of cancer risk can proceed no further than computation of the 50% risk to children of affected parents. The physician may then be able to advise a patient of his excess cancer risk, yet he must concede his or her inability to presently determine whether or not the individual in fact possesses the deleterious gene (and can therefore be expected with a higher degree of certainty to eventually develop cancer). Beyond suggesting that high risk relatives undergo frequent examination for early cancer signs and providing compassion and empathetic understanding, very little concrete assistance can be offered. In this context it is understandable that such barriers to cancer control as repression, fatalism, and even outright refusal to cooperate with physicians would occur.

For the family described herein and others in which reliable diagnostic risk indicators (markers) are lacking, the question remains: What should the relative roles of research and counseling be? In other words, at what point can the investigation of such families be considered so complete that the researchers are in a position to put their findings to work in a positive way for patient benefit? This is essentially a question of how much uncertainty the members of the family should be expected to bear regarding their own prognosis or that of their children.

Factors to be considered in making the decision to inform the family members (including the determination of what is to be revealed) include:

1. *The degree of rapport established with the individual members of the family.*

Willingness to cooperate in data collection has been found to be a good indicator of receptivity to our subsequent attempts to counsel. Refusal to assist in information gathering, despite encouragement by other relatives, reflects a more general unwillingness to heed suggestions pertaining to cancer control measures. At times an indirect approach, where the family physician is advised of pertinent findings, as he or she should be anyway, can be more successful in that the recalcitrant patient may respond more readily to advice from his or her own physician. Where the patient may well be transmitting the deleterious trait to his or her children, a more aggressive stance may be required since repression by the patient should not be allowed to endanger (even potentially) his or her offspring.

2. *Access by safe diagnostic procedures to high risk organs.*

Where, as in the subject family, a patient is at 50% risk for cancer of the colon, is it realistic to expect the patient to submit to indicated diagnostic procedures such as colonoscopy and/or barium enemas on an annual basis, especially where substantial travel and expense is involved? Such travel expense and loss of work time are rarely (if ever) covered under an insurance plan and exposure to radiation risk may make some diagnostic procedures counter-productive if carried out over a period of years.

An even more difficult situation presents itself in families prone to ovarian cancer. Not only is ovarian carcinoma an especially pernicious form of cancer, but the difficulty of safely diagnosing it at an early stage is an extremely perplexing problem. A prudent management decision in certain circumstances may be prophylactic oophorectomy. However, given the emotional factors involved in suggesting prophylactic oophorectomy to a woman of childbearing age, the need for sensitive counseling cannot be understated. For example, an attempt was made to counsel a woman from a family prone to carcinoma of the breast and ovary regarding the nature of her cancer risk and possible options available to her, including prophylactic oophorectomy (and bilateral mastectomy). Although the counseling was performed in a nondirective manner, her decision ultimately had to be based on the weighing of compelling physical and emotional considerations: the possibility of future child-bearing versus the risk for ovarian (or breast) carcinoma with high mortality. Of course, each factor had other considerations inextricably bound up with them, and although these considerations may have been subsidiary to this woman, they could well have taken on greater prominence in a woman already having a greater or lesser number of children, or one not married at all, or one who was more willing to risk eventual cancer, etc. Given the fact that all patients and counselees vary in the weight given to their individual factors, the counselor must fully develop and discuss each of them, based on his or her knowledge of responses by earlier patients or counselees. Such patients or counselees may have chosen or rejected prophylactic surgical intervention for reasons which may not have occurred to the person being counseled currently.

The well-intentioned family physician and/or genetic investigator might well decide that it is better to say nothing, rather than alarm a patient who would not be in a position to help himself or herself, despite an awareness of risk to a particular organ. The problem with such an approach is that the patient or counselee will have been alarmed by the very fact of the information gathering process. In our experience it has proven almost impossible to stimulate family members to provide needed research information without at some point alluding to the suspected familial nature of the cancer occurrences. Indeed, during the interview process with members of the subject family, we found that nearly all relatives already had some notion of the extent of cancer in the family, were aware that there might be some inherited predisposing factor involved, and further suspected that they personally were at high cancer risk.

3. *The importance of clarity and full disclosure.*

There is a well-known tendency for physicians to withhold certain information from patients due to the legitimate fear that the latter will misconstrue what is said or otherwise lack the capacity to participate prudently in the judgment process pertaining to the proper course of management. The choice may be to say nothing or to explain all the details in the hope that the patient or counselee would not misunderstand what factors or issues the physician was contemplating. Unfortunately, it cannot always be known whether the patient or counselee has understood the implications of what has been explained. Since familial cancer problems cannot be eradicated (except by restricting procreation or prophylactically removing a possibly healthy organ), due to present limitations in genetic engineering, the problem will exist in the family indefinitely. This is why it is essential to thoroughly explain the mode of genetic transmission (when known), age range of maximum risk, as well as early diagnostic and preventive measures (total prophylactic colectomy at diagnosis of familial polyposis coli or total prohpylactic colectomy in those patients who have had hemicolectomy for colon cancer of this familial variety).

An indispensible adjunct to a well-designed cancer education process is the presentation of pertinent findings to family physicians. This should take little time and will be appreciatively received. The family physicians who have been informed of the mode of transmission and clinical features of the syndrome will be able to provide invaluable follow-up. They will be able to respond in greater detail to patients' questions and pass pertinent information on to any subsequent physicians. The underlying consideration throughout is the fact that the family doctors will be able to more effectively convince the family members under their care that the condition is manageable if such management is indeed possible. This, of course, is one of the ultimate goals in genetic counseling.

Our clinical experience indicates that a nondirective counseling approach is most satisfactory (Lynch, 1969). The counselor must provide the patients (counselees) with an opportunity to have a satisfying verbal catharsis since this may be the first time in the patients' life that they have had an opportunity to discuss fully their concerns and reactions to the cancer issue in their family. This may become the most potent aspect of the genetic counseling process. A flexible approach will enable the patients to comprehend why they feel the way they do about the problem and may allow them to adopt a positive and psychologically adjusted role in management of the familial cancer susceptibility. In problems such as these, it is often advisable to counsel the spouse, children, and other available close relatives so that a more full comprehension of the problem can be achieved by those individuals who are or may be at increased cancer risk or who, like the spouse, are ego-involved with the problem.

The Physician and Genetic Counseling

SCOPE OF GENETIC COUNSELING

Any patient or relative who is concerned about the known or inferred risk for a disorder which has either a presumptive or proven genetic etiology should be given appropriate counseling. However, in order to accomplish this feat, considerable medical and genetic information must be available. If one couples the late age of onset and difficulty in arriving at a specific diagnosis short of histologic verification with variable gene penetrance, expressivity, and environmental influences, it is apparent that care and cautious deliberation must be exercised so that the patient or counselee is not given information based on erroneous or speculative risk figures. Furthermore, in the case of a life-threatening disease such as cancer, where diagnosis may be critical to survival and where preventive measures are sometimes possible, the physician must assume major responsibility in assuring that the best possible diagnosis and therapy are provided the patient and the family.

We view genetic counseling as embodying a total commitment to patient and family management, which, of course, considers the socio-psychological milieu as well as the medical problems of diagnosis, therapy, prognosis, and disposition. Unfortunately, some geneticists and physicians believe that "genetic counseling" implies solely the stereotyped quotation of simply derived statistical risks to the counselee. This is obviously a severely restricted approach. Indeed, it is totally inadequate! Genetic counseling involves total patient management and must be viewed with the same gravity as any medical problem requiring the establishment of a patient–physician relationship.

Dissemination of Genetic Risk Information

It is important for the counselor to recognize that risk information may be received and interpreted by the patient or counselee in a variety of ways depending upon intellectual capabilities, cultural background, and ego involvement with the problem at hand. The latter is usually determined by the individual's position in the pedigree; in other words, how closely the risk bears upon him or her and the immediate family. For example, the degree of ego involvement will vary between a spouse who has married into the family (not likely to contract the disease, but has children at high risk), and an individual who is affected or has an inordinately high risk for developing the particular disorder by virtue of having an affected parent.

The severity of the disease and its amenability to effective treatment or prevention will also have a major bearing on the acceptance of the genetic risk information. Pearn (1973) has discussed in some detail the events which influence the patient's subjective interpretation of risks which are offered in genetic counseling. People differ markedly in their attitude to genetic risk information; this variation appears to form a continuous spectrum ranging from extreme cautiousness and even hypochondriasis to blatant recklessness. However, attempts to qualify the propensity for risk acceptance as well as the particular individual's attitude toward quoted probabilities have to date been unsuccessful. Nevertheless, it is important that the genetic counselor estimate his or her counselee's interpretation of risk figures when they are given. This is important in that the counselor's responsibility is to be certain that meaningful communication of the particular risk is provided the counselee and that a reasonable understanding of the risk, including intellectual and emotional acceptance of the implications of such risk, be obtained. This obviously is the art of counseling and will determine in a major way the need for continued contact with the counselee where it is apparent that the individual has not yet attained a reasonable understanding and emotional acceptance of the newly described status.

The manner in which a risk figure is expressed to the counselees may have a major bearing on their interpretation of it. For example, if both parents are known to be heterozygotes for a recessive gene, then there are two possible ways of expressing the risk that they will have affected or unaffected children. It can be expressed as a one-in-four risk of the particular disease or trait occurring or it can be expressed as a three-to-one chance that the child will be normal. In the case of a couple who desperately desires to have a normal child, especially after they have lost one or more children from a fatal recessive disease, and when it is apparent that they are going to "try again," it might be well for the counselor to express the risk in terms of a three-to-one chance of their having a normal child. This may provide a certain measure of reassurance and comfort during the waiting period before they have another child. Similar expression of risk can be given for dominant disorders where it can be emphasized that the counselee has a 50% chance of having a *normal* child as opposed to a negative approach through emphasis upon the 50% risk for having an *affected* child.

According to Pearn, prior discussions of the risk situation may lead to an increased willingness on the part of the counselee to accept greater risks.

One of the problems in genetic counseling is to provide accurate information for persons who may have been grossly misinformed about genetic risks in the past. This is particularly difficult when they have been provided information by so-called "experts" such as other genetic counselors or physicians who themselves may for one reason or another have been misinformed. This results from the lack of a correct diagnosis; for example, a sporadic disease may have been interpreted as a genetic one or the previous counselor may not have been aware of the mode of genetic transmission of the particular disorder.

Divergent Responses to Risk Information

The strong desire for children is still a basic truism in our society. Of course, every parent wants to have healthy children. The desire to have children is present prior to the knowledge of the particular genetic counseling status of the parent. However, the counselor may find that the implications of the risk information may be contrary to the traditional beliefs and desires of the counselee. For this reason, in a cancer associated condition which is dominantly inherited, the responses of the counselees might include the following:

1. They may ignore the counseling risk information and have as many children as they wish

2. The counselees may have relatively few children, possibly one or two, accepting the genetic risk, but hoping that these will be in the 50% category of *unaffected* offspring. They may even be willing to accept the eventuality that one or even two of the children might be affected, but consider this risk satisfactory in light of advances in our preventive and diagnostic capabilities.

3. They may wish to forego having children and adopt instead.

4. In case of an affected male, he may wish to be sterilized and have artificial insemination provided for his wife. An affected female may simply elect to have a sterilization procedure.

These possibilities denote the situation which must be managed head-on by the counselor. Indeed, the counselor must be prepared to provide the counselees with sufficient information about all of the possible alternatives which may result from their decision-making process. Most important in genetic counseling, the counselor must avoid imposing his or her own views and feelings on the counselees. Only maturity and experience will aid the counselor in this very difficult area.

Heritable Cancer Syndromes Amenable to Genetic Counseling

Approximately 161 (9%) of the 866 known single-gene traits (and the 1010 others that are suggestive but have inconclusive evidence of Mendelian behavior) (McKusick, 1976) include malignant or benign neoplastic lesions as either a primary feature or as a frequent, occasional, or rare complication (Mulvihill, 1975).

Physical Stigmata in Hereditary Precancerous Disorders

Genetic counseling is aided appreciably by the presence in the patient of physical stigmata (sometimes recognizable at birth) that denote a particular hereditary precancerous syndrome. The readily apparent physical signs might also alert members of the family, allowing them to be cognizant of the fact that they are or may be affected with the family "trait." In certain situations, relatives may make the correlation between these physical signs and cancer susceptibility.

When present, characteristic cutaneous signs (e.g., the *cafe' au lait* spots and or neurofibromas of von Recklinghausen's neurofibromatosis, the neuromas of the oral mucosa or conjunctiva in the multiple mucosal neuroma syndrome and the increased freckling in xerederma pigmentosum) have been used in genetic counseling as a basis for explaining the inherited precancerous diathesis. It allows the counselor to draw attention to tangible evidence of the disorder and to correlate this with a predisposition to cancer. Patients generally comprehend the issue of inheritance more clearly when they are able to identify the reproducibility of the stigmata in other members of the family and associate these signs with the high risk of cancer.

Gardner's Syndrome

Devic and Bussy (1912) described a lady who manifested sebaceous cysts of the scalp, subcutaneous lipomas, osteomas of the mandible, and multiple polyposis coli. This association of cutaneous and osseous lesions was shown by Gardner to constitute an hereditary precancerous syndrome (Gardner, 1955, 1963). Since these early reports, numerous occurrences of this disease have been documented. Its mode of inheritance has been consistently shown to be due to a simple autosomal dominant factor. McKusick (1962) has suggested that this syndrome is the result of a single gene that is distinct from that of simple familial polyposis coli.

Diagnostic features may vary from patient to patient and from family to family. Sebaceous cysts of the skin represent the most common soft-tissue tumor in this syndrome; large cysts around the face and neck are particularly characteristic. Benign osteomas are the more frequently observed bone abnormalities in Gardner's syndrome. These consist of dense, bony proliferations that may be variable in size and may be found in all areas of the skeletal system. Localized cortical thickening of the long tubular bones is also a common osseous abnormality in Gardner's syndrome families (Chong, Piatt, Thomas, & Watne, 1968). The frontal bone is the most frequent site of osteoma in the skull. Dental abnormalities, including supernumerary and unerupted teeth, have been described in this syndrome

Any patient who develops soft-tissue tumors and/or osteomas should be carefully evaluated for the possible presence of polyposis of the colon. Should a patient have a positive family history of Gardner's syndrome, the patient should then be considered at particularly high risk for colon cancer. Just as in familial polyposis coli, nearly 100% of patients with Gardner's syndrome will develop adenocarcinoma of the colon by age 50. Therefore, once diagnosis of Gardner's syndrome is established and polyposis coli has been recognized, the patient should be immediately prepared psychologically for prophylactic colectomy. One always asks, "What is the earliest age at which a colectomy should be performed?" This is a difficult question because of the drastic nature of this form of prevention. However, it should be remembered that colon cancer has been identified in 16 patients under the age of 15 who have manifested this syndrome. Another patient (Moore, Kupchik, Marcon, & Somchek, 1971) manifested five synchronous colon carcinomas at age 14 and 4 years later developed adenocarcinoma of the ampulla of Vater. Thirteen years following his initial colon surgery he developed a transitional cell carcinoma of the bladder.

A variety of cancers have been described in Gardner's syndrome. Some of these may be found to be firmly associated with the disease. Tumors have included anaplastic carcinomas of the mandible, fibrous tumors of the parotid glands, thyroid carcinoma, and a variety of sarcomas. Thus, the patient must be advised that prophylactic colectomy will only remove the highest risk target site, and the possibly associated tumors of other sites will still have to be considered, requiring life-long cancer surveillance.

Multiple Nevoid Basal Cell Carcinoma Syndrome

The triad of jaw cysts, skeletal anomalies, and multiple nevoid basal cell carcinomas constitute the multiple nevoid basal cell carcinoma syndrome. More than 250 individuals with the syndrome have been described and the spectrum of anomalies has increased considerably. These now include ovarian fibroma, lympho-mesenteric cysts, intracranial calcification, possible parathormone hyporesponsiveness, occasional occurrences of medulloblastoma, and a variety of lesser associated anomalies. The facies in certain patients may show distinguishing characteristics including tempo-parietal bossing, well-developed supraorbital ridges, ocular hypertelorism, mild mandibular prognathism, and possibly ophthalmoplegia.

Skin is the primary target organ for cancer and the characteristic lesions are multiple nevoid basal cell carcinomas that may occur exceedingly early in the life of a patient, as early as the second year. Lesions may occur in both exposed and unexposed cutaneous areas. There is marked variation in the expression of these skin lesions and in certain patients skin lesions may even be absent. The skin lesions are often numerous and may appear as tiny, flesh-colored to brownish dome-shaped papules, soft nodules, or flat plaques that vary in diameter from 1 mm to 1 cm. The commonly affected sites in order of decreasing frequency include the face and neck, back and thorax, abdomen, and upper extremities. Other skin lesions have included cysts, comedones, *cafe' au lait* pigmentation, hirsutism, and multiple pigmented nevi. Interestingly, small indentations of the skin of the palm or soles, referred to as palmarplantar pits, have been noted. Some investigators consider these palmarplantar pits to be a pathognomonic sign of the syndrome. This disorder is inherited as an autosomal dominant.

Genetic counseling should include careful admonition about signs of malignant transformation in the cutaneous lesions so that prompt therapy can be given the patient. Because the lesions are so frequent and the skin so susceptible to malignant transformation, radiation is not advised. Topical application of 5-fluorouracil and surgical excision are the treatments of choice.

Testicular Feminization Syndrome

The testicular feminization syndrome (TFS), while rare, nevertheless provides a useful model for genetic counseling. Emotional implications are profound in this disorder.

The typical patient with this syndrome is a genetic male (XY chromosome complement) who has a female habitus and whose axillary and pubic hair are scanty or absent; female external genitalia with variable stages of under-development of labia are manifested. There will be a blind-ending vagina that is usually adequate for sexual relations. Patients may have a rudimentary uterus and gonads (testes) that may be intra-abdominal or may be found along the course of the inguinal canal. These testes are comprised primarily of seminiferous tubules and are usually characterized by the absence of spermatogenesis though they frequently have a marked increase in interstitial cells. Thus, these patients have outward manifestations of a female, and unless intervention in the form of an attempt to change the sexual identification is made, they will manifest the psychosexual orientation of a female. Indeed, they often marry and may enjoy a normal sex life (Lynch, 1976).

Family studies reveal an inheritance pattern with transmission through the maternal line consistent with either a sex-linked recessive or male sex-limited autosomal dominant mechanism. To date, delineation of the true genetic mechanism has not been accomplished (Stenchever, Ng, Jones, & Jarvis, 1969).

Of importance for purposes of this chapter is the fact that individuals with the syndrome have an inordinately high risk for development of carcinoma of the testes. Although Morris and Marash (1963) found only one patient with cancer below the age of 20, they did find 11 cases (or 22%) in patients over 30 years of age. Other estimates of cancer rates include 5% in the study of Jones and Scott (1958), and 8% in the study of Hauser (1963). It is difficult, however, to establish a true incidence of cancer in patients with TFS since many of these patients have been treated with prophylactic gonadectomy at an early age.

Of the testicular cancers, the most common is seminoma (Cornet, Loubiere, & Serres, 1971), although other tumors including teratocarcinoma and embryonal cell carcinoma have been described (Gans & Rubin, 1962; Scully, 1970).

Genetic counseling in this disorder requires compassion, understanding, and considerable ingenuity on the part of the counselor since the sexual identity of the patient is usually well-established and, as mentioned, some of these patients may already be married and enjoying a satisfying sexual relationship. One school of thought would have the findings (XY status) presented to the patient in a completely straightforward manner. Although each counselor must make his own value judgment regarding the amount of information to be divulged, we feel that little can be gained by disclosing the fact that the patient is genotypically a male versus the harm that could ensue psychologically.

Counseling should consider the cancer risk to the patient's gonads. The issue of prophylactic gonadectomy should be discussed in detail. The timing of prophylactic gonadectomy is important, though controversial. Some authors have suggested the need for immediate gonadectomy even in prepubertal patients (Gans & Rubin, 1962) while others have been reluctant to advise prophylactic gonadectomy for any of these patients (Hauser, 1963).

National Familial Cancer Registry System

The proposed National Familial Cancer Registry System could be a vehicle for ultimate resolution of the mentioned dichotomy between investigation of poorly understood syndromes and management of particular patients who exhibit well-documented disorders. Its combination of systematic documentation of family and medical histories and computerized storage for rapid retrieval of the latest diagnostic and counseling procedures would enable family physicians to know which of their patients are members of high risk kindreds and how to most effectively deal with them. For example, when members of families with polyposis coli syndromes are ascertained, their physician may need only be informed of the patient's genetic risk status and receive materials pertaining to differential diagnosis and management. Literature describing the more reliable modes of treatment, such as colectomy with ileo-rectal anastomosis, would then be provided. In a kindred that exhibits a familial disorder where cancer risk is empirically derived, as in certain occurrences of carcinoma of the breast, stomach, colon, prostate, and endometrium, a slightly different approach would be required. Until more definite ascertainment of a possible precancerous state is possible, physicians caring for members of such families should be informed about current research in the area and urged to follow their patients carefully with particular attention given to high risk target organs. In this case, the compilation of a number of families would constitute primarily a research tool, facilitating the acquisition of information. Yet, the information compiled could be readily utilized for its service capability when advances occur, which would allow it to be applied for the benefit of these already ascertained families.

The genetic counselor has an important moral, if not legal obligation to the patient's family (Lynch & Lynch, 1976), particularly when a treatable or preventable disorder is segregating. Thus, it would seem narrowminded and imprudent to diagnose familial polyposis coli in an individual patient, offer advice on prophylactic colectomy, and yet ignore the possibility of this same disease in the patient's several brothers, sisters, or children, all of whom are at 50% risk for its development. It is mandatory that the genetic counselor view the particular hereditary disorder in the context of the whole family (Tips & Lynch, 1963) and provide advice and a management program that will encompass and eventually benefit all of these high risk relatives.

Summary and Conclusions

Genetic counseling in cancer raises certain problems that are quite unique. One of the most important issues is the long latent period of this disease in that many of the patients have already married and procreated prior to the onset of cancer. In many respects this is similar to the hereditary ataxias, Huntington's Chorea, myotonia dystrophica, and other hereditary disorders characterized by a late age of onset. Unlike these noncancerous hereditary diseases, cancer is an extremely common condition. When appropriate age corrections are made, one may predict that approximately 25% of the population will be afflicted with this disease, and about 15% of the population will ultimately expire from cancer. The ordinarily high frequency of this disease may therefore obfuscate the genetic issue since patients with commonly occurring lesions such as carcinoma of the breast, endometrium, lung, and colon may aggregate in a particular family by chance alone or as a result of shared nongenetic or environmental carcinogenic exposures.

Certain forms of hereditary cancer may be prevented. For example, autosomal dominantly inherited colon cancer may be controlled in familial polyposis coli and related syndromes through prophylactic colectomy. Medullary thyroid carcinoma and pheochromocytoma may be controlled in Sipple's syndrome and the multiple mucosal neuroma syndrome through exceedingly early diagnosis (aided by calcitonin assay and syndrome identification). Thus, the genetic counselor may promote life-saving measures in families prone to carcinoma of a variety of anatomic sites by identifying those in need of and amenable to early detection and in certain circumstances, prophylactic surgery.

We have emphasized the importance of providing insight to the counselee and to those relatives who are at high risk for cancer. Genetic counseling can therefore meet some of the broader facets of cancer control in high risk kindreds, a factor which should significantly increase its worth from a public health standpoint.

Finally, in a real sense of the word, genetic counseling is both patient and family management with an emphasis upon disease control.

A decade ago we suggested the "Ten Commandments" for genetic counseling. These appear to be particularly applicable to the cancer issue and are repeated here in order to embellish the philosophy and objectives of genetic counseling as perceived by the authors.

1. Genetic counseling is an integral part of the management of the patient with genetic disease, the responsibility for which ideally should be assumed by the family physician.

2. The counselor must never make decisions for the patient regarding marriage, children, and other important personal issues. These decisions are the patient's responsibility and only he or she should exercise this right.

3. The genetic counselor must take meticulous care to insure the accuracy of diagnosis in hereditary disease in that ramifications of such a diagnosis may profoundly affect the entire family unit.

4. The counselor must look beyond the individual patient and be

concerned with eliciting support for the medical welfare of other affected members of the kindred.

5. The genetic counselor must constantly remember that the presence of hereditary disease in the family may promote strong emotional reaction among unaffected as well as affected members of the kindred; the counselor must do everything possible to alleviate this emotional stress.

6. The genetic counselor must strive to effectively dispel unfavorable impressions and irrational responses by members of the community against individuals with certain "grotesque" mental and physical hereditary disorders. The physician will usually be in a favorable position in the community to institute a positive educational program toward this goal.

7. The genetic counselor must study all aspects of the natural history of hereditary diseases, so that when needed he or she may effectively mobilize paramedical personnel and community resources to help the patient and the family.

8. Care must be taken to exclude extragenetic factors as being of etiologic importance. Should a nongenetic factor be the major cause of disease, as in rubella syndrome, parents must be reassured and thoroughly informed that the disorder in their midst is not genetic, should this be the case.

9. Hearsay evidence of disease in relatives of the affected proband should be verified whenever possible; effort extended in this direction will be highly rewarding in the long run.

10. The genetic counselor will be in a favorable position to study variations in known hereditary disorders as well as to uncover "new" hereditary diseases. The counselor should make every effort to report scientific observations to his or her colleagues.

References

Brasher, P. H. Clinical and social problems associated with familial intestinal polyposis. *American Medical Association Archives of Surgery*, 1954, 69, 785–796.

Chong, C. H., Piatt, E. D., Thomas, K. E., & Watne, A. L. Bone abnormalities in Gardner's Syndrome. *American Journal of Roentgenology*, 1968, 103, 645–652.

Cornet, L., Loubiere, R., & Serres, J. J., et al. Gonophoric male pseudohermaphroditism with abdominal cryptorchidism and cancer of the testis: A case of seminoma associated with a testicular feminization syndrome. *Chirurgie*, 1971, 97, 64–73.

Day, E. The patient with cancer and the family. *New England Journal of Medicine*, 1966, 274, 883–886.

Devic, A., & Bussy, N. M. Un cas de polypose adenomateuse generalise' a tout l'intestin. *Archives des Maladies de l'Appareil Digestif*, 1912, 6, 278–299.

Gans, S. L., & Rubin, C. L. Apparent female infants with hernias and testes. *American Journal of Diseases of Children*, 1962, 104, 114–118.

Gardner, E. J. Mendelian pattern of dominant inheritance for a syndrome including intestinal polyposis, osteomas, fibromas and sebaceous cysts in a human family group. *American Journal of Human Genetics*, 1955, 2, Medelione, L. Gedda, ed.: pp. 321–329.

Hauser, G. A. Testicular feminization. In *Intersexuality*. L. Overzier, (Ed). London: London Academic Press, 1963.

Jones, H. W., Jr., & Scott, U. N., (Eds.). *Hermaphroditism, gentic anomalies and related endocrine disorders*. Baltimore: Williams and Wilkins, 1958.

Krush, A. J., Krush, T. P., & Lynch, H. T. Psycho-social factors in a family with a disfiguring genetic trait. *Psychosomatics*, 1965, 6, 391–396.

LeFevre, H. W., Jr., & Jacques, T. G. Multiple polyposis in an infant of four months. *American Journal of Surgery*, 1951, 81, 90–91.

Lipkin, M., & Deschner, E. Early proliferative changes in intestinal cells. *Cancer Research*, 1976, 36, 2665–2668.

Lynch, H. T. *Dynamic genetic counseling for clinicians*. Springfield, Illinois: Thomas Co., 1969.

Lynch, H. T. *Skin, heredity and malignant neoplasms*. Flushing, N.Y.: Medical Examination Publishing Co., pp. 299,. 1972.

Lynch, H. T. Genetic counseling and cancer. In Lynch, H. T. (Ed.), *Cancer genetics*. Springfield, Illinois: Thomas Co., 1976.

Lynch, H. T. Management and control of familial cancer. In Mulvihill, J. J. (Ed.) *Genetics of human cancer*, New York: Raven Press, 1977.

Lynch, H. T., Guirgis, H. A., Albert, S., Brennan, M., Lynch, J., Kraft, C., Pocekay, D., Vaughns, C., & Kaplan, A. Familial association of carcinoma of the breast and ovary. *Surgery, Gynecology, and Obstetrics*, 1974, 138, 717–724.

Lynch, H. T. Guirgis, H. A., Brodkey, F., Lynch, J., Maloney, K., Rankin, L., Mulcahy, G. Genetic heterogeneity and familial carcinoma of the breast. *Surgery, Gynecology, and Obstetrics*, 1976, 142, 693–699.

Lynch, H. T. & Krush, A. J. The cancer family syndrome and cancer control. *Surgery, Gynecology, and Obstetrics*, 1971, 123, 247–250.

Lynch, P. M. & Lynch, H. T. Medical-legal aspects of familial cancer. *Journal Legal Medicine*, 1976, 4, 10–16.

Lynch, P. M., Lynch, H. T., Harris, R. E., Lynch, J. F. & Guirgis, H. A. Heritable colon cancer and solitary adenomatous polyps. *Proc. 3rd International Symposium on Detection and Prevention of Cancer*, New York: Marcel-Dekker Co.

McKusick, V. A. Genetic factors in intestinal polyposis. *Journal of the American Medical Association*, 1962, 182, 271–277.

McKusick, V. A. *Mendelian inheritance in man*. Baltimore: Johns Hopkins Univ. Press, 1966.

Moore, T. L., Kupchik, H. Z., Marcon, V., & Somchek, N. Carcinoembryonic antigen assay in cancer of the colon and pancreas and other digestive tract disorders: a preliminary report. *Lahey Clinic Foundation Bulletin*, 1971, 20, 85–88.

Morris, J. M., & Maresh, V. B. Further observations on the syndromes "testicular feminization". *American Journal of Obstetrics and Gynecology*, 1963, 87, 731–748.

Mulvihill, J. Congenital and genetic diseases. In J. F. Fraumeni, (Ed), *Persons at high risk of cancer: An approach to cancer etiology and control*. New York: Academic Press, 1975.

Pearn, J. H. Patients' subjective interpretation of risks offered in genetic counseling. *Journal of Medical Genetics*, 1973, 10, 129–134.

Scully, R. E. Gonodoblastoma: A review of 74 cases. *Cancer*, 1970, 25, 1340–1356.

Stenchever, M. A., Ng, A. B. P., Jones, G. K., & Jarvis, J. A. Testicular feminization syndrome: Chromosomal, histologic and genetic studies in a large kindred. *Obstetrics and Gynecology*, 1969, 33, 649–657.

Tips, A. L. & Lynch, H. T. The impact of genetic counseling upon the family milieu. *Journal of the American Medical Association*, 1963, 184, 183–186.

WHO Expert Committee on Human Genetics. *Technical Report Series*, 1969, 416, 5–23.

Subject Index

A

Abandonment, 9, 23, 202–203, 206, 214

Abortion, 7, 27, 29–30, 108, 109–112, 193
consequences of, 29–30, 111–112, 193
meaning of, 29–30, 193

Activity–passivity, 2–3, 24, 54–55, 76, 86, 211–212

Ambivalence, 26, 29, 59, 61, 73, 86–87

Amniocentesis, 1, 7, 27–28, 107–113, 123–124
decision making, 107–113, 123–124
fear of procedure, 100
limitations of procedure, 109
psychological meaning, 108
safety of procedure, 107
waiting for results, 28, 110

Anchoring, 44, 67

Anger, 47, 71, 81, 111, 131, 132, 157, 206–209
response of professionals to, 157–158

Anxiety, 27–28, 38–39, 83, 108, 120, 192

Archetypes, 29

Avoidance responses, 8, 47, 155–156, 159, 164

B

Behavior control, 59–61

Behavior technology, 5, 59

Birth defects,
frequency, 109 *see also* Genetic disorders, frequency

Body image, 27, 155–156, 164, 187, 214–215

C

Cancer, 9, 221–239
of the colon, 224–229
medical management, 225–226, 229
predicative tests, 225–226
delay phenomenon, 224
Familial Cancer Registry System, 236–237
family, effects on, 223
Gardner's syndrome, 233–234
characteristics, 233–234
medical management, 234
multiple nevoid basal cell carcinoma syndrome 234–235
characteristics, 234–235
medical management, 235
Precancerous disorders, 233